Recent Advances in Alternative Medicine

Edited by Cengiz Mordeniz

Published in London, United Kingdom

Recent Advances in Alternative Medicine
http://dx.doi.org/10.5772/intechopen.1000427
Edited by Cengiz Mordeniz

Contributors
Benio Kibushi, Amel Elbasyouni, Stephen Wilson Kpordze, Hadil Suliman Hussein, Oumarou Soro, Samuel Mulondo, Jonas Nshimirimana, Tekeba Sisay Melese, Le Quynh Mai, Jie Yang, Liying Liu, Xiaoyan Zheng, Jingwen Zhang, Yuanyuan Lai, Dorly de Freitas Buchi, Edvaldo S. Trindade, Carolina C. de Oliveira

First published in London, United Kingdom, 2023 by IntechOpen
IntechOpen is the global imprint of INTECHOPEN LIMITED, registered in England and Wales, registration number: 11086078, 5 Princes Gate Court, London, SW7 2QJ, United Kingdom

British Library Cataloguing-in-Publication Data
A catalogue record for this book is available from the British Library

Additional hard and PDF copies can be obtained from orders@intechopen.com

Recent Advances in Alternative Medicine
Edited by Cengiz Mordeniz
p. cm.
Print ISBN 978-1-83769-700-7
Online ISBN 978-1-83769-699-4
eBook (PDF) ISBN 978-1-83769-701-4

Meet the editor

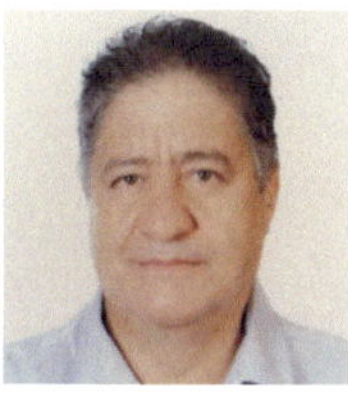

Professor Dr. Cengiz Mordeniz is part of the Medical Faculty, Department of Anesthesiology and Intensive Care and Pain Medicine, Tekirdag Namik Kemal University, Turkey. He also works at the Traditional and Complementary Medicine Center of the University Hospital, performing digital homeopathy, hirudotherapy, cupping therapy, apitherapy and apipuncture, and ozone therapy. He is interested in vibrational and informational medicine to predict pathologies in energetic biofields in advance and modulate them through frequency therapies.

Contents

Preface

Modern medicine has for a long time ignored traditional and alternative methods. In the last decade, the World Health Organization, European Union, and other international and national health authorities have begun to view alternative medicine in a more positive light and issue new regulations to integrate these methods into modern medical practice. Thus, new trials and research on alternative medical methods have gained popularity. This book presents a comprehensive overview of alternative medicine.

Chapter 1 focuses on motion, electromyography, and biofeedback. Recently, health has been redefined as wellness and lifestyle, in which regular exercise plays a key role. Because a sedentary lifestyle has negative impacts on health, the musculoskeletal structure of the human body and its flexibility are gaining more importance. The future direction of health may be vibrational or energy medicine, which detects pathologies at early stages in the bioenergetic field of the human body and rebalances the body's energy field to restore health.

Current medical applications are mostly somatic. However, biofield therapies that use energy fields to restore health are gaining popularity. Chapter 2 discusses informational communication from the body as it relates to cancer. In the human body, there are dynamic informational channels functioning in the infrared spectral range. This informational system starts from the cell itself and continues to other bodily systems. In the informational age, current medical applications focusing on the somatic body should go expand further to bioinformatics and informational medicine.

Chapter 3 discusses homeopathy, which is part of the trend towards personalized, holistic medicine. The chapter examines the benefits and success of the homeopathic approach.

Acupuncture has been used for centuries and is the most popular traditional method of alternative medicine. Chapter 4 analyzes acupuncture's use in modern medicine in the field of reproductive technology.

Chapter 5 examines the use of traditional Vietnamese food spices for medical purposes.

Medicine is constantly being redefined as medical consumers gravitate towards more personalized and holistic approaches to maintaining their health. Lifestyle management instead of reliance on pharmaceuticals is the future of modern medicine.

As such, this book focuses on alternative medicine, presenting new approaches to health and wellness that consider people's biopsychosocial and spiritual perspectives.

Cengiz Mordeniz
Medical Faculty,
Department of Anesthesiology and Intensive Care and Pain Medicine,
Tekirdag Namik Kemal University,
Tekirdag, Turkiye

Chapter 1

Electromyography Biofeedback to Improve Dynamic Motion

Benio Kibushi

Abstract

Electromyography biofeedback (EMG-BF) has been used to train muscle activation or relaxation but the application of EMG-BF to improve dynamic motion (e.g., walking or pedaling) is open to investigation. This chapter deals with an introduction to our previous work and the latest research we are working on. In our previous study, we investigated whether auditory EMG-BF is effective in improving muscle co-contraction. Unfortunately, we found that individual EMG-BF does not immediately improve muscle co-contraction during pedaling. To improve muscle co-contraction by EMG-BF, it may be necessary to convert muscle activation into muscle co-contraction. In our latest study, we investigated whether visual EMG-BF is effective in stabilizing walking. We found that EMG-BF during normal walking partially stabilizes the center of mass acceleration. Finally, based on our research findings, I will discuss the construction of an EMG-BF system that can contribute to the improvement of dynamic movements.

Keywords: muscle activity, walking, pedaling, kinematics, stability

1. Introduction

Biofeedback has been utilized as a rehabilitative approach to facilitate normal movement patterns. Humans have sensory receptors such as muscle spindles and tendon spindles, which engage in feedback control based on the information received from sensory receptors. Patients can access physiological data that would typically unnoticed in real-time by biofeedback. This aims to enhance the acquisition of normal movement patterns.

In this chapter, the focus is on electromyography biofeedback (EMG-BF). One of the functions of muscles is to move joints through contraction. Muscle contraction occurs when electrical signals from the brain reach the muscles via nerves. As electrical activity arises during muscle contraction, the measurement of electrical activity during muscle contraction on the surface of the skin has been employed as a means to examine the dynamics of muscle contraction. Obtaining electrical signals during muscle contraction is known as an electromyogram (EMG). Electromyography biofeedback (EMG-BF) involves converting the EMG into a visual or auditory feedback signal, establishing a novel feedback system, and contributing to the reacquisition of movements or learning new movements. Electromyography biofeedback (EMG-BF) is employed to enhance the activity of weakened or paralyzed muscles, as well as to alleviate tension in spastic muscles.

In this chapter, I will begin by briefly introducing previous studies on the effects of EMG-BF. A more comprehensive review of EMG-BF can be found in the works of Giggins et al. [1] and Huan et al. [2]. Furthermore, I will present our research on the utilization of EMG-BF for improving dynamic movements. Finally, based on our research findings, I will discuss the construction of an EMG-BF system that can contribute to the improvement of dynamic movements.

1.1 Static EMG-BF

Previous research on EMG-BF has been addressed by various experimental tasks. Among these tasks, there were simple movements unrelated to daily activities, such as users adjusting specific parameters while in a static state [3–6]. Huang et al. [2] referred to this as "static biofeedback" [2]. Static EMG-BF also proves useful in rehabilitation. For example, applying static EMG-BF in rehabilitation after knee joint surgery leads to improvements in knee joint range of motion [7], peak torque during knee extension [8], and activation level of the knee extensor muscles [9]. However, static EMG-BF might have limited effectiveness. This is because the improvement is observed when the purpose is to alter the activity of the target muscle itself or when the target muscle is directly related to joint control. Moreover, several studies and reviews on static EMG-BF have not demonstrated significant contributions to the recovery of motor function [3, 10, 11]. For instance, Wolf et al. [11] used static EMG-BF to suppress the activity of antagonist muscles of the elbow extensor and activate the agonist's muscle. However, this method prevented stroke patients from fully extending their elbows during a reaching task and caused muscle co-contraction during coordinated movements [11]. Additionally, applying static EMG-BF to the lower limbs of hemiparetic patients had no impact on functional gait [3]. Therefore, static EMG-BF might have limited effectiveness in promoting the recovery of motor function [12].

1.2 EMG-BF for improving walking abilities

The effectiveness of EMG-BF in improving walking abilities remains a subject of debate. According to a systematic review, it was concluded that EMG-BF does not have a significant effect on joint range of motion, functional capacity, stride, or walking speed following stroke [13]. However, several studies have reported positive results. For instance, adding EMG-BF to conventional exercise programs significantly reduced the usage time of walking aids in patients who underwent surgery for arthroscopic partial meniscectomy, compared to those who received only conventional exercise training [14]. Particularly, in children with cerebral palsy, many positive outcomes have been reported [15–17]. For example, EMG-BF targeting the tibialis anterior during walking led to improvements in symmetry and greater ankle power for push-off in children with cerebral palsy [15]. Furthermore, when children with cerebral palsy used EMG-BF, it resulted in improved foot clearance during the swing phase of walking and the acquisition of new abilities for contraction and relaxation of the anterior tibialis muscle [16]. Thus, opinions on whether EMG-BF improves walking abilities are divided. Such contradictions might depend on the specific type of EMG-BF utilized. Earlier, it was explained that static EMG-BF might have limited effectiveness in promoting the recovery of motor function. Therefore, static EMG-BF might not be suitable for improving walking. Consequently, it is believed that EMG-BF directly related to walking movement would be effective in enhancing walking performance.

2. Auditory EMG-BF for improving muscle co-contraction

2.1 Introduction

The inhibition of smooth movement often arises from muscle co-contraction occurring between agonist and antagonist muscles. Effectively improving muscle co-contraction could potentially contribute to promoting motor learning. However, there is limited research demonstrating the adjustment of muscle coordination patterns through EMG-BF. Torricelli et al. [18] reported a change in synchronous muscle activity patterns by providing biofeedback for the tibialis anterior muscle during pedaling [18]. Nevertheless, the effects of EMG-BF on muscle co-contraction remain unclear.

Biofeedback systems primarily use visual or auditory feedback [13]. Previous studies showed auditory EMG-BF reduced frontalis muscle activation, unlike visual EMG-BF [19]. Additionally, auditory feedback facilitated higher sensory integration than visual feedback [20]. Moreover, motor learning through the auditory feedback achieved a higher motor learning effect [20] and higher accurate posture control ability [21] even after removing auditory feedback, but the visual feedback did not. Faster auditory reaction times to stimuli [22] suggest auditory EMG-BF may prompt more immediate muscle adjustments than visual EMG-BF. Thus, we hypothesized that auditory EMG-BF enhances muscle co-contractions. We aim to investigate its effectiveness in improving muscle co-contraction and contribute to more effective EMG-BF methodologies' development.

2.2 Auditory EMG-BF system

The participants had EMG electrodes attached to them to record muscle activity. The vastus lateralis (VL) and the semitendinosus (ST) on the right side were the muscles tested for feedback. Using an analog data acquisition system, the EMG data was transferred into a personal computer and monitored via a specially designed LabVIEW program. The EMG data, which was recorded at 1000 Hz, was then processed in real-time through full-wave rectification and smoothing via the weighted moving average.

During the determining a threshold, participants engaged in a one-minute pedaling session at the workload assigned for adjustment or measurement tasks. The VL and ST were rectified and smoothed in order to establish each muscle's peak value. Thresholds were defined when the normalized EMG amplitude exceeded 5% of the maximum amplitude during pedaling compared to the amplitude at rest, a method determined through preliminary experiments. The threshold was progressively altered, and participants have queried whether the beeping corresponded to their muscle activation timing. We established the lowest threshold that could consistently produce an appropriate sound. Beep frequencies were designated as 400 Hz for VL and 800 Hz for ST.

2.3 Experimental procedures

Six women and seven men participated in this study (women: age 25 ± 3 years, height 160 ± 5 cm, body weight 53 ± 4 kg; men: age 25 ± 3 years, height 171 ± 5 cm, body weight 69 ± 9 kg, [mean ± standard deviation]).

Pedaling was chosen for the experiment due to its simplicity and the co-contraction phase it includes. Skill level correlates with muscle co-contraction during pedaling, with cyclists displaying less co-contraction than triathletes [23]. Improving co-contraction may require increasing agonist activation while decreasing antagonist activities.

The experiment followed this order: instruction, initial threshold adjustment for EMG-BF system, adaptation to clipless pedals and EMG-BF system, workload determination, second threshold adjustment, and kinematics and EMG measurements (**Figure 1**). Participants pedaled for 20 minutes to adapt to the clipless pedal and the EMG-BF system [24]. The threshold adjustment was necessary as the EMG-BF system beeped when muscle activation exceeded a certain threshold, chosen from a study finding pure tone sounds acceptable for athletes during rowing [25].

In the study, the workload was determined based on heart rate monitoring. During adaptation, cadence and workload were adjusted to keep heart rates between 100 and 120 bpm. Beep sounds were used for muscle activity feedback, aiming to reduce overlap. After a 10-minute rest, the workload for measurement was set so that the heart rate maintained around 150 bpm at 80-cadence. The workload increased by 20 W/min until 150 bpm could no longer be maintained. The relative workload was selected based on heart rate, considering both sexes participated. Average workloads for women and men were 123 ± 26 W and 176 ± 26 W, respectively. A 10-minute rest followed workload determination. During measurement tasks, participants pedaled for 90 seconds at 80-cadence with a determined workload.

Four feedback conditions during measurement tasks were: no-feedback (NFB), VL feedback (VLFB), ST feedback (STFB), and both VL and ST feedback (VL-STFB). In addition to NFB, the need to compare individual EMG-BF as in the previous study [4] and EMG-BF agonist-antagonist muscles was assumed. In VL-STFB, we asked participants not to overlap the beep sound.

2.4 Measurement and analysis

In order to capture the movements associated with pedaling, reflective markers were affixed to the right pedal and crank. A four-camera 3D motion capture system operating at 100 Hz was used to record these position coordinate values. The topmost position of the pedal stroke was identified as a crank angle of zero, defining one complete cycle as the movement from one topmost position to the next.

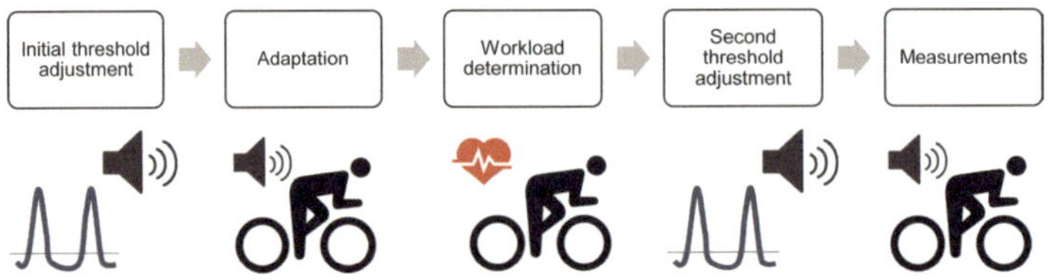

Figure 1.
Experimental procedures.

Alongside the VL and ST, EMG signals from the rectus femoris (RF) and long head of the biceps femoris (BF) were also measured to study the co-contraction of muscles involved in hip flexion-extension. The EMG signals from RF and BF were recorded at a frequency of 1000 Hz. The EMG signals were high-pass filtered (20 Hz) with a zero-lag fourth-order Butterworth filter to remove motion artifacts. Thereafter, the EMG signals were demeaned, digitally rectified, and low-pass filtered at 15 Hz with a zero-lag fourth-order Butterworth filter. These low-pass filtered signals were then time interpolated over a single cycle of motion to conform to a normalized 200-point time base. Each muscle's activity was normalized to its peak activity recorded across all conditions.

Normalized EMG data were used to estimate the co-contraction index (COI), which represents the degree of simultaneous activation between agonist and antagonist's muscle. The COI of the hip flexor-extensor (RF-BF) and knee extensor-flexor (VL-ST) was assessed using the following (Eq. 1) [26, 27]:

$$COI = \frac{2 \times Common\ Area}{(area\ EMG_1 + area\ EMG_2)} \times 100 \tag{1}$$

where $area\ EMG_1$ and $area\ EMG_2$ represent the integral of the sum of agonist and antagonist EMG data. $Common\ Area$ represents the common area between agonist and antagonist EMG data (**Figure 2**).

After confirming normal data distribution, repeated measurement of ANOVA was applied to determine the difference in COI among the different conditions. The results with a p-value < 0.05 were considered significant.

2.5 Auditory EMG-BF did not improve muscle co-contraction

We observed no significant difference in COIs among the conditions (**Table 1**).

Contrary to our hypothesis, auditory EMG-BF does not improve muscle co-contractions. This might be because our auditory EMG-BF system might have some problems. We suggest an idea for improving muscle co-contraction by auditory EMG-BF.

Initially, let us discuss how muscle activity did not see enhancement. We hypothesized that the regulation of muscle relaxation during pedaling presents more challenges because modulating force while muscles are relaxed is tougher than when they are generating force [28]. Nevertheless, unsuitable patterns were noted in both the relaxation of antagonist's muscles and the activation of agonist muscles. In a qualitative observation, the ST was found to be active between 270 and 360 degrees of the crank angle in this study. This insufficient relaxation of antagonist muscle might cause high COI of VL-ST around the top dead center. According to Candotti et al. [23], the BF activation in triathletes was only seen from 0 to 180 degrees of the crank angle,

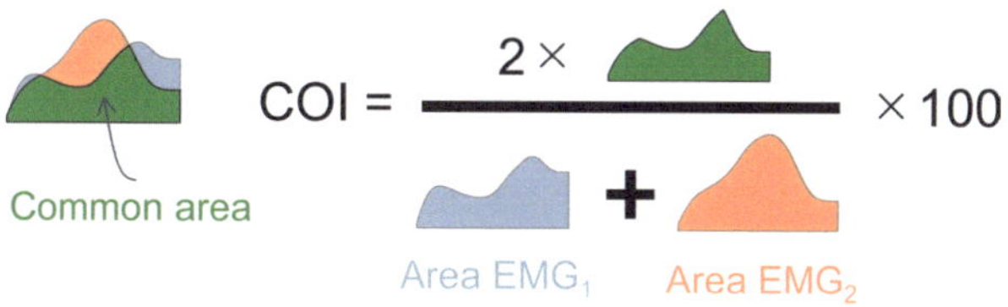

Figure 2.
Illustration of COI.

	Average ± SD	*p*-value
COI of VL-ST		
NFB (%)	47.8 ± 13.1	0.83
VLFB (%)	48.8 ± 12.1	
STFB (%)	48.1 ± 13.0	
VL-STFB (%)	49.2 ± 12.0	
COI of RF-BF		
NFB (%)	54.1 ± 11.3	0.32
VLFB (%)	56.5 ± 9.8	
STFB (%)	53.5 ± 12.0	
VL-STFB (%)	55.9 ± 11.0	

Table 1.
COI of VL-ST and RF-BF.

while cyclists showed activity beyond the bottom dead center, leading to the inference that reduced BF activation contributes to a higher COI in triathletes. In our study, the ST and BF activations beyond the bottom dead center were not significant under all conditions. This insufficient activation of the agonist's muscle could possibly lead to a high COI of VL-ST around the bottom dead center.

2.6 Future issues for auditory EMG-BF to improve muscle co-contraction

Now, let us consider the issues related to the system. The lack of improvement in muscle co-contraction observed in our study might be due to the suboptimal setup of the EMG-BF system. Specifically, the EMG-BF system may not be fully capable of translating muscle co-contraction. According to Peres et al. [4], the most accurate muscle activation timing could be estimated when the feedback sound's pitch and loudness were adjusted [4]. In our study, we maintained constant loudness and varied pitches to make it easier for the participants to discern different muscle activities. When questioned about their muscle activity perception during the EMG-BF system adjustment, the participants reported that they could discern individual muscle activities as well as the overlap of multiple muscle activities. Nevertheless, modifying the feedback sound's pitch and loudness might have been a more suitable approach.

Besides the matters of pitch and loudness, the differing feedback sounds of EMG could potentially result from cognitive overload. In this study, participants identified both the activation and relaxation of agonist-antagonist muscles either as a single beep or a combination of different beeps. Previous research indicates that the simultaneous processing of multiple pieces of biomechanical output information can decrease pedaling endurance performance due to information overload [29]. The auditory feedback from two muscles could indeed lead to the presentation of multiple pieces of information. Nonetheless, it is generally accepted that multimodal stimuli are perceived more accurately and quickly than unimodal stimuli [30, 31]. Sigrist et al. [32] suggested that if the workload in one sensory modality is high, augmented feedback should be provided in another modality or in a multimodal manner. This could prevent cognitive overload, and therefore, might enhance motor learning. Considering this viewpoint, auditory information about the timing of individual muscle activities might be inadequate for modifying muscle co-contraction. For instance, in our study, there was no feedback on the intensity of muscle co-contraction. To enhance the feedback, the visualization of the COI might be a solution. Consequently, it may be necessary to transform the signals of individual agonist and antagonist muscle activation into a co-contraction signal. Moreover, a system that combines visual feedback of COI with sound feedback that adjusts pitch and loudness based on muscle co-contraction signals may be more effective.

2.7 Conclusion

We examined the effectiveness of using beep sounds with EMG-BF to enhance muscle co-contraction. Our results indicated that EMG-BF did not improve muscle co-contraction during pedaling. In order to boost muscle co-contraction via EMG-BF, there might be a need to transform the signal of individual agonist and antagonist muscle activation into a co-contraction signal. Our conclusion is that instant improvement of muscle co-contraction during pedaling is challenging using individual EMG-BF.

3. Visual EMG-BF for stabilizing walking

3.1 Introduction

Normal walking is typified by kinematic stability, evidenced by the steady patterns of head and lumbar acceleration and the reduction of variability in trunk motion from stride to stride at a regular walking pace [33, 34]. The root mean square (RMS) of upper body acceleration is a frequently employed measure of kinematic stability, with a higher RMS signifying instability in circumstances like walking on uneven surfaces for healthy young adults or associating with an increased risk of falls in elderly individuals [35, 36].

Rhythmic auditory stimulation (RAS), which employs a metronome, has been implemented in physical therapy to correct irregular walking, thus enhancing cadence and stride length, and decreasing stride time variability in patients with Parkinson's disease [37–40]. However, RAS with a fixed tempo could potentially cause unstable walking in healthy adults [40, 41], indicating the possible necessity for non-stationary auditory stimulation.

Electromyography biofeedback (EMG-BF) provides another non-stationary stimulation technique, which could affect walking stability due to the direct influence of muscle activity on joint force application [42, 43]. Previous research has shown that EMG-BF enhances walking ability in stroke patients and children with cerebral palsy [15, 17, 44, 45]. The goal of the current study is to build upon these findings by investigating if EMG-BF improves walking stability in healthy adults, positing that it reduces the RMS of the center of mass acceleration (RMS-CoM$_{acc}$). This study represents the inaugural exploration of the impact of EMG-BF on walking stability in healthy adults.

3.2 Experimental procedure and analysis

The study involved the participation of five women and seven men (women; age: 23 $\pm$ 5 years, height: 160 $\pm$ 3 cm, body mass: 54 $\pm$ 7 kg, men; age: 21 $\pm$ 1 years, height:

169 ± 3 cm, body mass: 66 ± 4 kg [mean ± standard deviation]). To gather kinematic data, reflective markers were positioned on 24 body landmarks. These coordinate positions were captured using a three-dimensional motion tracking system equipped with 10 cameras, operating at a frequency of 100 Hz. We recorded EMG data from four muscles in the right lower limb and trunk, specifically, the soleus (SOL), tibialis anterior (TA), vastus lateralis (VL), and semitendinosus (ST).

The participants in this study were assigned two tasks: a maximum voluntary contraction (MVC) task and a walking task. The MVC task involved four main movements: ankle plantarflexion, ankle dorsiflexion, knee extension, and knee flexion. Prior to recording the measurements, participants practiced each MVC task and the RMS of the EMG data was computed around the maximum value for each MVC task. The walking task had participants walk on a treadmill with or without EMG biofeedback. The biofeedback conditions included soleus (SOLBF), tibialis anterior (TABF), semitendinosus (STBF), and a no biofeedback scenario (NBF). Before measurements were collected, participants had a practice session on the treadmill. The EMG-BF system would make a beeping sound if the muscle activity went above a certain threshold based on the MVC. Each EMG-BF had three different thresholds, and the order of the conditions was randomized. During EMG-BF, participants aimed to sustain a consistent beep sound tempo.

Three-dimensional RMS-CoM_{acc} was used to gauge walking stability, computed from the second-order derivative of the center of mass position (anteroposterior [AP], vertical [VT], mediolateral [ML]). Statistical comparison was conducted among the RMS-CoM_{acc} across biofeedback conditions. For each biofeedback condition, only one threshold condition was extracted for comparison. This was because the RMS-CoM_{acc} minimizing threshold condition varied among participants and within the same participant, depending on the direction. Data normality was confirmed with the Shapiro-Wilk test before conducting repeated measure ANOVA. Significance was determined at $p < 0.05$, with marginally significant results considered at $0.05 \leq p < 0.10$.

3.3 Auditory feedback of soleus reduces RMS-CoM_{acc} in AP and VT direction

We found that the RMS-CoM_{acc} in both the AP and VT directions was significantly lower in the SOLBF condition than in the NBF condition (**Figure 3**), indicating that the direction in which the RMS-CoM_{acc} decreases depends on the muscle being used for biofeedback. An earlier study showed that the SOL and lateral gastrocnemius muscles are responsible for decelerating the trunk backward during the loading response phase and propelling the trunk forward during the propulsion phase [46]. In addition, the SOL and lateral gastrocnemius muscles are primarily responsible for the vertical acceleration of the trunk [46]. Since the SOL plays a crucial role in creating both AP and VT trunk acceleration, SOLBF might decrease the RMS-CoM_{acc} in both AP and VT directions. Moreover, in terms of comfort, SOLBF seems to be the most suitable biofeedback condition. When asked about the biofeedback condition that was easiest for modulating their muscle activation, most participants chose SOLBF. The SOL has a relatively distinct monophasic waveform, unlike the TA and ST. The waveform's shape could be related to the ease of modulating muscle activation. The decrease in RMS-CoM_{acc} as a result of EMG-BF could be related to both the biomechanical contributions to trunk acceleration and usability.

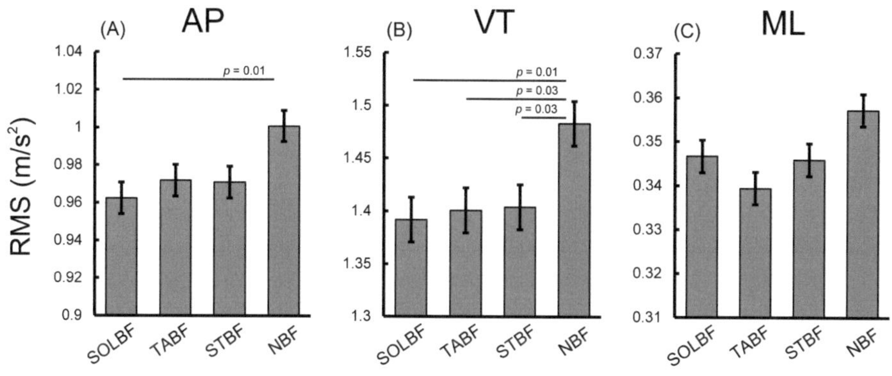

Figure 3.
Average RMS-CoM$_{acc}$ in AP, VT, and ML direction.

3.4 Auditory EMG-BF did not reduce RMS-CoM$_{acc}$ in ML direction

We noted that EMG-BF did not decrease the RMS-CoM$_{acc}$ in the ML direction (**Figure 3**). Previous studies suggest that the link between trunk acceleration in the AP and VT directions is stronger than the connections between the ML and AP directions and between the ML and VT directions [47]. This could suggest that the modulation of trunk acceleration in the ML direction operates somewhat independently. This independent modulation in the ML direction could be connected to the constant RMS-CoM$_{acc}$ in the ML direction during EMG-BF. Another possible explanation for the stable RMS-CoM$_{acc}$ in the ML direction is that we may not have chosen a muscle involved in moving the body in the ML direction for EMG-BF. We chose the ankle plantar flexor, ankle dorsiflexor, and knee flexor for EMG-BF, muscles primarily involved in moving the body in the VT or AP directions. To reduce the RMS-CoM$_{acc}$ in the ML direction, we might need to select hip abductor or adductor muscles for EMG-BF.

3.5 Conclusion

We aimed to find out if EMG-BF improves walking stability in healthy adults. While EMG-BF did have a slight reducing effect on RMS-CoM$_{acc}$, this effect was minimal. Notably, biofeedback of the ankle plantar flexor managed to decrease both anteroposterior and vertical RMS-CoM$_{acc}$. We concluded that biofeedback of the ankle plantar flexor can marginally stabilize the anteroposterior and vertical center of mass acceleration during walking.

4. Summary and general discussion

This chapter deals with an introduction to our previous work and the latest research we are working on. In our previous study, we investigated whether auditory EMG-BF is effective in improving muscle co-contraction. Unfortunately, we found that individual EMG-BF does not immediately improve muscle co-contraction during pedaling. To improve muscle co-contraction by EMG-BF, it may be necessary to convert muscle activation into muscle co-contraction. In our latest study, we investigated whether visual EMG-BF is effective in stabilizing walking. We found that EMG-BF in soleus during normal walking partially stabilizes the center of mass acceleration.

Through two studies, insights have been obtained regarding the requirements for constructing an EMG-BF system capable of enhancing dynamic movements. These insights include:

- Converting muscle activity into discernible signals
- Selecting the most relevant muscles associated with the desired stabilized movements as feedback targets
- Adjusting the threshold individually for auditory feedback

While research on static EMG-BF has been conducted for a long time, there remains ample room for exploration regarding EMG-BF specifically aimed at improving dynamic movements. Consequently, it is necessary to construct a system based on the aforementioned insights and validate its effectiveness in enhancing various dynamic movements other than pedaling and walking.

Acknowledgements

This work was supported by the TOBE MAKI Scholarship Foundation (Grant number: 19-JC-002), JSPS KAKENHI (Grant number: 21K17627), and CAINZ Digital Innovation Foundation.

Conflict of interest

The author declares no conflict of interest.

Author details

Benio Kibushi
Graduate School of Human Development and Environment, Kobe University, Kobe, Japan

*Address all correspondence to: kibushi.b@ruby.kobe-u.ac.jp

References

[1] Giggins OM, Persson UM, Caulfield B. Biofeedback in rehabilitation. Journal of Neuroengineering and Rehabilitation. 2013;**10**:60

[2] Huang H, Wolf SL, He J. Recent developments in biofeedback for neuromotor rehabilitation. Journal of NeuroEngineering and Rehabilitation. 2006;**3**(1):1-12

[3] Bradley L, Hart BB, Mandana S, Flowers K, Riches M, Sanderson P. Electromyographic biofeedback for gait training after stroke. Clinical Rehabilitation. 1998;**12**(1):11-22

[4] Peres SC, Verona D, Nisar T, Ritchey P. Towards a systematic approach to real-time sonification design for surface electromyography. Displays. 2017;**47**:25-31

[5] Davis PJ. Electromyograph biofeedback: Generalization and the relative effects of feedback, instructions, and adaptation. Psychophysiology. 1980; **17**(6):604-612

[6] Nielsen DH, Holmes DS. Effectiveness of EMG biofeedback training for controlling arousal in subsequent stressful situations. Biofeedback and Self-Regulation. 1980; **5**(2):235-248

[7] Xie YJ, Wang S, Gong QJ, Wang JX, Sun FH, Miyamoto A, et al. Effects of electromyography biofeedback for patients after knee surgery: A systematic review and meta-analysis. Journal of Biomechanics. 2021;**120**:110386

[8] Draper V, Ballard L. Electrical stimulation versus electromyographic biofeedback in the recovery of quadriceps femoris muscle function following anterior cruciate ligament surgery. Physical Therapy. 1991;**71**(6): 455-464

[9] Kirnap M, Calis M, Turgut AO, Halici M, Tuncel M. The efficacy of EMG-biofeedback training on quadriceps muscle strength in patients after arthroscopic meniscectomy. The New Zealand Medical Journal. 2005; **118**(1224):U1704

[10] Kohlmeyer KM, Hill JP, Yarkony GM, Jaeger RJ. Electrical stimulation and biofeedback effect on recovery of tenodesis grasp: A controlled study. Archives of Physical Medicine and Rehabilitation. 1996;**77**(7):702-706

[11] Wolf SL, Catlin PA, Blanton S, Edelman J, Lehrer N, Schroeder D. Overcoming limitations in elbow movement in the presence of antagonist hyperactivity. Physical Therapy. 1994;**74** (9):826-835

[12] Kimmel HD. The relevance of experimental studies to clinical applications of biofeedback. Biofeedback Self Regul. 1981;**6**(2):263-271

[13] Woodford H, Price C. EMG biofeedback for the recovery of motor function after stroke. Cochrane Database of Systematic Reviews. 2007;**2007**(2): CD004585

[14] Akkaya N, Ardic F, Ozgen M, Akkaya S, Sahin F, Kilic A. Efficacy of electromyographic biofeedback and electrical stimulation following arthroscopic partial meniscectomy: A randomized controlled trial. Clinical Rehabilitation. 2012;**26**(3):224-236

[15] Colborne GR, Wright FV, Naumann S. Feedback of triceps surae EMG in gait of children with cerebral palsy: A controlled study. Archives of

Physical Medicine and Rehabilitation. 1994;**75**(1):40-45

[16] Bolek JE. A preliminary study of modification of gait in real-time using surface electromyography. Applied Psychophysiology and Biofeedback. 2003;**28**(2):129-138

[17] Dursun E, Dursun N, Alican D. Effects of biofeedback treatment on gait in children with cerebral palsy. Disability and Rehabilitation. 2004;**26**(2):116-120

[18] Torricelli D, De Marchis C, D'Avella A, Tobaruela DN, Barroso FO, Pons J. Reorganization of muscle coordination underlying motor learning in cycling tasks. Frontiers in Bioengineering and Biotechnology. 2020;**8**:1-17

[19] Alexander AB, French CA, Goodman NJ. A comparison of auditory and visual feedback in biofeedback assisted muscular relaxation training. Psychophysiology. 1975;**12**(2):119-123

[20] Ronsse R, Puttemans V, Coxon JP, Goble DJ, Wagemans J, Wenderoth N, et al. Motor learning with augmented feedback: Modality-dependent behavioral and neural consequences. Cerebral Cortex. 2011;**21**(6):1283-1294

[21] Hasegawa N, Takeda K, Mancini M, King LA, Horak FB, Asaka T. Differential effects of visual versus auditory biofeedback training for voluntary postural sway. PLoS One. 2020;**15**(12): e0244583

[22] Kohfeld DL. Simple reaction time as a function of stimulus intensity in decibels of light and sound. Journal of Experimental Psychology. 1971;**88**(2): 251-257

[23] Candotti CT, Loss JF, Bagatini D, Soares DP, da Rocha EK, de Oliveira ÁR, et al. Cocontraction and economy of triathletes and cyclists at different cadences during cycling motion. Journal of Electromyography and Kinesiology. 2009;**19**(5):915-921

[24] Mornieux C, Stapelfeldt B, Collhofer A, Belli A. Effects of pedal type and pull-up action during cycling. International Journal of Sports Medicine. 2008;**29**(10):817-822

[25] Dubus G. Evaluation of four models for the sonification of elite rowing. Journal on Multimodal User Interfaces. 2012;**5**(3–4):143-156

[26] Souissi H, Zory R, Bredin J, Gerus P. Comparison of methodologies to assess muscle co-contraction during gait. Journal of Biomechanics. 2017;**57**: 141-145

[27] Winter DA. Biomechanics and Motor Control of Human Movement. 4th ed. Hoboken, NJ: Wiley; 2009

[28] Ohtaka C, Fujiwara M. Force control characteristics for generation and relaxation in the lower limb. Journal of Motor Behavior. 2019;**51**(3):331-341

[29] Bayne F, Racinais S, Mileva K, Hunter S, Gaoua N. Less is more—Cyclists-Triathlete's 30 min cycling time-trial performance is impaired with multiple feedback compared to a single feedback. Frontiers in Psychology. 2020;**11**:1-11

[30] Doyle MC, Snowden RJ. Identification of visual stimuli is improved by accompanying auditory stimuli: The role of eye movements and sound location. Perception. 2001;**30**(7): 795-810

[31] Giard MH, Peronnet F. Auditory-visual integration during multimodal object recognition in humans: A

behavioral and electrophysiological study. Journal of Cognitive Neuroscience. 1999;**11**(5):473-490

[32] Sigrist R, Rauter G, Riener R, Wolf P. Augmented visual, auditory, haptic, and multimodal feedback in motor learning: A review. Psychonomic Bulletin & Review. 2013;**20**(1):21-53

[33] Latt MD, Menz HB, Fung VS, Lord SR. Walking speed, cadence and step length are selected to optimize the stability of head and pelvis accelerations. Experimental Brain Research. 2008; **184**(2):201-209

[34] Dingwell JB, Marin LC. Kinematic variability and local dynamic stability of upper body motions when walking at different speeds. Journal of Biomechanics. 2006;**39**(3):444-452

[35] Menz HB, Lord SR, Fitzpatrick RC. Age-related differences in walking stability. Age and Ageing. 2003;**32**(2): 137-142

[36] Senden R, Savelberg HHCM, Grimm B, Heyligers IC, Meijer K. Accelerometry-based gait analysis, an additional objective approach to screen subjects at risk for falling. Gait & Posture. 2012;**36**(2):296-300

[37] Thaut MH, Abiru M. Rhythmic auditory stimulation in rehabilitation of movement disorders: A review of current research. Music Perception. 2010;**27**(4):263-269

[38] McIntosh GC, Brown SH, Rice RR, Thaut MH. Rhythmic auditory-motor facilitation of gait patterns in patients with Parkinson's disease. Journal of Neurology, Neurosurgery, and Psychiatry. 1997;**62**(1):22-26

[39] Arias P, Cudeiro J. Effects of rhythmic sensory stimulation (auditory, visual) on gait in Parkinson's disease patients. Experimental Brain Research. 2008;**186**(4):589-601

[40] Hausdorff JM, Lowenthal J, Herman T, Gruendlinger L, Peretz C, Giladi N. Rhythmic auditory stimulation modulates gait variability in Parkinson's disease. European Journal of Neuroscience. 2007;**26**(8):2369-2375

[41] Roerdink M, Daffertshofer A, Marmelat V, Beek PJ. How to sync to the beat of a persistent fractal metronome without falling off the treadmill? PLoS One. 2015;**10**(7):e0134148

[42] Kang HG, Dingwell JB. Dynamics and stability of muscle activations during walking in healthy young and older adults. Journal of Biomechanics. 2009;**42** (14):2231-2237

[43] Kang HG, Dingwell JB. Effects of walking speed, strength and range of motion on gait stability in healthy older adults. Journal of Biomechanics. 2008; **41**(14):2899-2905

[44] Aiello E, Gates DH, Patritti BL, Cairns KD, Meister M, Clancy EA, et al. Visual EMG biofeedback to improve ankle function in hemiparetic gait. In: Annual International Conference of the IEEE Engineering in Medicine and Biology 27th Annual Conference-Proceedings; Shanghai. Institute of Electrical and Electronics Engineers Inc.; 2005. pp. 7703-7706

[45] Jonsdottir J, Cattaneo D, Regola A, Crippa A, Recalcati M, Rabuffetti M, et al. Concepts of motor learning applied to a rehabilitation protocol using biofeedback to improve gait in a chronic stroke patient: An A-B system study with multiple gait analyses. Neurorehabilitation and Neural Repair. 2007;**21**(2):190-194

[46] Neptune RR, Kautz SA, Zajac FE. Contributions of the individual ankle plantar flexors to support, forward progression and swing initiation during walking. Journal of Biomechanics. 2001; **34**(11):1387-1398

[47] Kavanagh JJ, Morrison S, Barrett RS. Coordination of head and trunk accelerations during walking. European Journal of Applied Physiology. 2005;**94** (4):468-475

Chapter 2

The Crosstalk between Phytotherapy and Bioinformatics in the Management of Cancer

Amel Elbasyouni, Stephen Wilson Kpordze, Hadil Suliman Hussein, Oumarou Soro, Samuel Mulondo, Jonas Nshimirimana and Tekeba Sisay Melese

Abstract

Natural products and medicinal plants have been extremely important contributors to the field of drug development due to their ability to bind to and change cellular targets that have been linked to cancer. On the other hand, when it comes to the quest for alternative treatments for cancer, bioinformatics and databases are of critical importance to the field of cancer research. The knowledge of drug-target interactions, the prediction of therapeutic efficacy and side effects, the identification of novel drug targets and the repurposing of current medications are all made easier by computer-aided drug design and network pharmacology. Through the use of bioinformatics, researchers are able to get a more in-depth understanding of the biology behind cancer and speed up the process of developing plant-based therapy options that are effective, safe, affordable and available. In this chapter, we provide a comprehensive review of computer-aided drug design and network pharmacology together with their importance in plant-based drug discovery in the era of cancer.

Keywords: cancer, therapy, plant-based, bioinformatics, drug discovery

1. Introduction

Worldwide, cancer is a major contributor to mortality rates and a major bottleneck to extending the human lifespan. Due to population ageing and growth, changes in the prevalence and distribution of cancer risk factors and socioeconomic development, the global burden of cancer incidence and mortality is increasing with 19.3 million new cases and 10 million deaths [1]. According to GLOBOCAN 2020, female breast cancer remains the most frequently occurring with 2,261,419 new cases (11.7%), followed by lung, prostate, nonmelanoma of the skin, colon stomach, liver, rectum and cervical [1]. Tobacco, alcohol consumption, high body mass index, low physical activity, endocrine disruptors, diet, socioeconomic status, hygiene and infections are the major extrinsic risk factors for cancerogenesis, whereases genomic signatures and cancer-specific mutations predispose to malign transformation and tumour development and progression [2–8].

Cancer development and progression are multistep processes. Fourteen hallmarks have been identified as cancer signatures, and have been relevant to understand its complexity and mechanism. These hallmarks include maintenance of proliferative signalling and an uncontrolled capacity of replication and proliferation, evading growth regulators, impaired regulation at the genomic level, evading the immune system, immortality, resistance to apoptosis and cell death mechanisms, maintained inflammation, polymorphic microbiome, senescence, genome instability and mutations in genes of predisposition, impaired metabolomics and hypoxia, angiogenesis, plasticity and invasion and metastasis [9].

Cancer genesis and its development mechanisms are linked to impaired signalling pathways due to driver and/or passenger mutations [10]. The Ras-ERK and PI3K-Akt signalling pathways are the major oncogenic pathways leading to uncontrolled proliferation, cell death resistance, metabolism alteration and migration, if consecutively active. Other pathways promoting the hallmarks of abnormal cells include Notch, NF-κB, Wnt/β-catenin and Hedgehog.

Conventional treatment regimens include radiotherapy, surgery, hormone-based therapy, chemotherapy and targeted therapy [11]. However, they are associated with many side effects, treatment resistance and failure, tumour relapse and metastasis. Therefore, there is an immediate need to develop and promote safe anti-cancer drug alternatives and integrate them into the routine clinical medicine. Plant-based traditional medicine is used worldwide as a first-stop therapy for the treatment and prevention of many diseases, including malaria, asthma and cancer [12–14]. Thus, there is a growing demand for serious scientific inquiry into the phyto-chemicals responsible for the activities of these plants. Currently, there are over 3000 plant species with confirmed anticancer properties [15], including Abrus precatorius, Albizzia lebbeck, Alstonia scholaries, Anacardium occidentale, Asparagus racemose, Boswellia serrata, Erthyrina suberosa, Euphorbia hirta, Gynandropis pentaphylla, Nigella sativa, Peaderia foetida, Catharanthus roseus, Picrorrhiza kurroa and Withania somnifera against various tumours. Interestingly, plant-derived secondary metabolites and their analogues have been already approved and commercialised due to their anti-cancer effectiveness and less toxicity (vincristine, paclitaxel, docetaxel...) compared to synthetic therapeutics associated with side effects, non-specificity and drug resistance [12, 15–19].

Unfortunately, research and development of new anti-cancer therapeutics is highly expensive (2 to 10 billion USD) [20]. In addition to the high cost, therapeutics are failing when brought to the clinical trials due to the high complexity and heterogeneity of cancer biology, plasticity and drug resistance [21]. Despite the sluggish pace of anticancer medication development, a number of approaches are worth exploring. New anticancer medications and the development of clinical paradigms around the world may 1 day benefit from an improved understanding of tumour heterogeneity and complexity.

Fortunately, the conventional drug research and development pipeline has been significantly speeded up, and the cost is reduced *via* integrating computational approaches and bioinformatics to provide more specific, cheaper, more effective and safer plant-based alternatives to cancer therapeutics [17, 22–27]. In this chapter, we aim to provide an explanation of the main computational approaches enhancing the area of plant-based anti-cancer drug research, development and discovery. We will discuss the pipeline of computer-aided drug design, and network pharmacology in order to promote the integration of medicinal plants and phytotherapy in the clinical oncology for a better management of cancer.

2. Computer-aided drug design

Structure-based strategy relies on the known three-dimensional structure of the proteins to define the interaction effect between bioactive compounds and the corresponding receptors to trigger therapeutic effects [28]. Biomolecular spectroscopic technologies such as X-ray crystallography and nuclear magnetic resonance spectroscopy (NMR) have improved our structural understanding of drug targets [29–32]. Hence, structure-based design can provide critical insights into new drug design, development and discovering and optimising initial lead compounds [33]. Novel and powerful, this computational strategy promotes medication discovery that is quicker, cheaper and more effective [34]. The following diagram provides an insight into the steps involved in structure-based drug design (**Figure 1**).

The first step is to choose a protein target with a known three-dimensional structure and involvement in a disease pathway [35]. A small molecule drug requires a binding site on the target. Getting the protein's three-dimensional structure is the next move. X-ray crystallography, NMR and other methods can be used for this purpose. The protein's structure can be utilised to locate locations where small-molecule medicines might bind. Molecular docking software, which estimates how tiny molecules might attach to the protein, can be used to examine these locations. In order to find small molecule compounds that bind to a target protein with high affinity and specificity after the binding site has been determined, a library of compounds can be screened [36]. This can be achieved through the use of either high-throughput screening techniques or virtual screening, or both. Compounds that fare well in the first round of screening go on to have their potency, selectivity and other drug-like qualities enhanced in subsequent rounds of testing [37]. Lead optimisation is the process of improving a compound's performance by altering the compound's chemical make-up. Molecular docking and dynamic simulation can be used to guide further optimisation [38]. The compounds that show the most promise go through *in vitro* and *in vivo* testing to determine their safety and effectiveness. This requires evaluating the drugs' pharmacokinetic and pharmacodynamic properties through testing in animal models. At last, the most promising chemicals are put through human clinical trials to determine whether or not they are safe and effective for use.

Available databases used for each step of the structure-based strategy are mentioned in the following table (**Table 1**).

In contrast to structure-based drug design, ligand-based drug design relies on the discovery of novel compounds with similar or enhanced biological activity by analysing the structural and physicochemical features of a ligand or a library of small molecules. **Figure 2** provides the steps involved in ligand-based drug design approach. Finding a target protein that is essential in cancer progression or development is the first step in ligand-based drug design. Followed by molecular docking process, where it is necessary to have either the 3D structure of the target protein or a homology model that might serve as a starting point [39]. After that, a library of ligands is compiled that have been shown to have biological activity against the target protein. The information in the database can come from either direct experimentation or from existing public sources in databases [39]. The binding mechanisms and affinities of the ligands to the target protein are predicted using a molecular

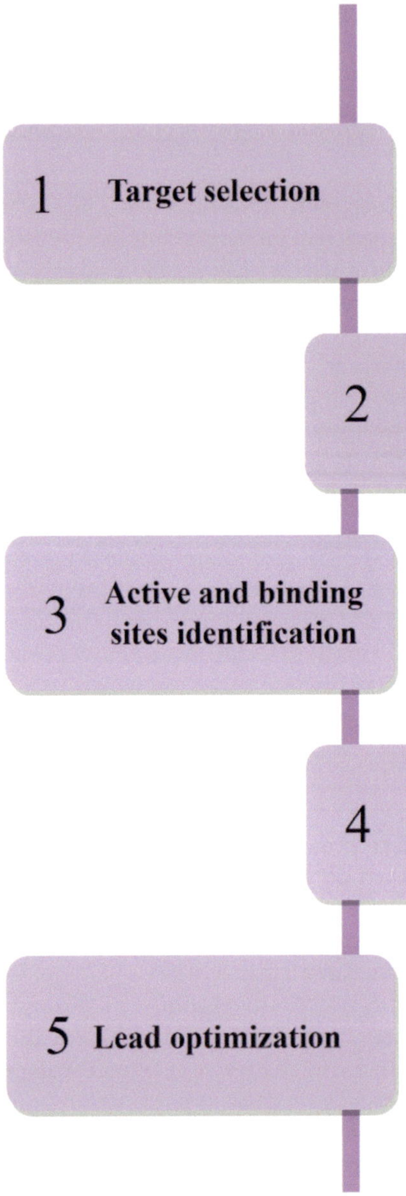

Figure 1.
Structure-based drug design flowchart.

docking programme. Drug discovery often uses molecular docking as it enables to visually analyse binding modes before making decisions [40]. After the ligands have been docked into the protein's binding site, the resultant complexes are evaluated according to their expected binding energies and interactions with the protein [38]. Predicted binding affinity, specificity and other physicochemical parameters are used to rank and filter the docked ligands. The best ligands are chosen for more study [41]. Computational chemistry techniques are then used to fine-tune the chosen ligands in order to increase their binding affinity, specificity and drug-like characteristics. Synthesis and experimental testing of the optimised ligands' biological

Step	Database	Link
Target selection	The Cancer Genome Atlas (TCGA)	https://www.cancer.gov/ccg/research/genome-sequencing/tcga
	cBioPortal	https://www.cbioportal.org/
	Cancer Genome Interpreter	https://www.cancergenomeinterpreter.org/home
	Cancer Cell Line Encyclopedia (CCLE)	https://sites.broadinstitute.org/ccle/
	DrugBank	https://go.drugbank.com/
3D structure retrieval	Protein Data Bank (PDB)	https://www.rcsb.org/
	RCSB Ligand Explorer	http://ligand-expo.rcsb.org/
	SWISS-MODEL	https://swissmodel.expasy.org/
	ModBase	https://modbase.compbio.ucsf.edu/
	Structural Classification of Proteins (SCOP)	https://scop.mrc-lmb.cam.ac.uk/
Active and binding sites identification	Catalytic Site Atlas (CSA)	https://www.ebi.ac.uk/thornton-srv/m-csa/
	BindingDB	https://www.bindingdb.org/rwd/bind/index.jsp
	Protein Data Bank (PDB)	https://www.rcsb.org/
	Conserved Domain Database (CDD)	https://www.ncbi.nlm.nih.gov/cdd/
	HOMSTRAD	https://mizuguchilab.org/homstrad/
Ligands/small molecules & Lead optimisation	ZINC Database	https://zinc.docking.org/
	PubChem	https://pubchem.ncbi.nlm.nih.gov/
	ChEMBL	https://www.ebi.ac.uk/chembl/
	DrugBank	https://go.drugbank.com/
	BindingDB	https://www.bindingdb.org/rwd/bind/index.jsp

Table 1.
Major databases used in structure-based drug design.

activities follow. Preclinical and clinical investigations are conducted on the optimised ligands to determine their efficacy and safety. The findings are used to hone the process for ligand-based drug creation and boost the precision and dependability of computational approaches.

The ligand-based drug design strategy is a useful method for discovering novel compounds that are both highly potent and selective against a target protein. To guarantee the anticipated ligands have the requisite pharmacological properties and can be converted into successful therapies, thorough validation and optimisation are necessary.

Rapidly dividing cancer cells are the primary targets of unspecific chemotherapeutic medications. However, certain normal cells are also affected, leading to the adverse side effects of major chemotherapeutics. Targeted cancer therapies inhibit the development and the progress of cancer by targeting certain proteins/molecular abnormalities that are unique to each tumour. Currently, two types of targeted medicines are developed: small molecule inhibitors and monoclonal antibodies. The small molecules attenuate the impaired kinases and abnormally overactivated signalling pathways, whereas monoclonal antibodies block extracellular proteins.

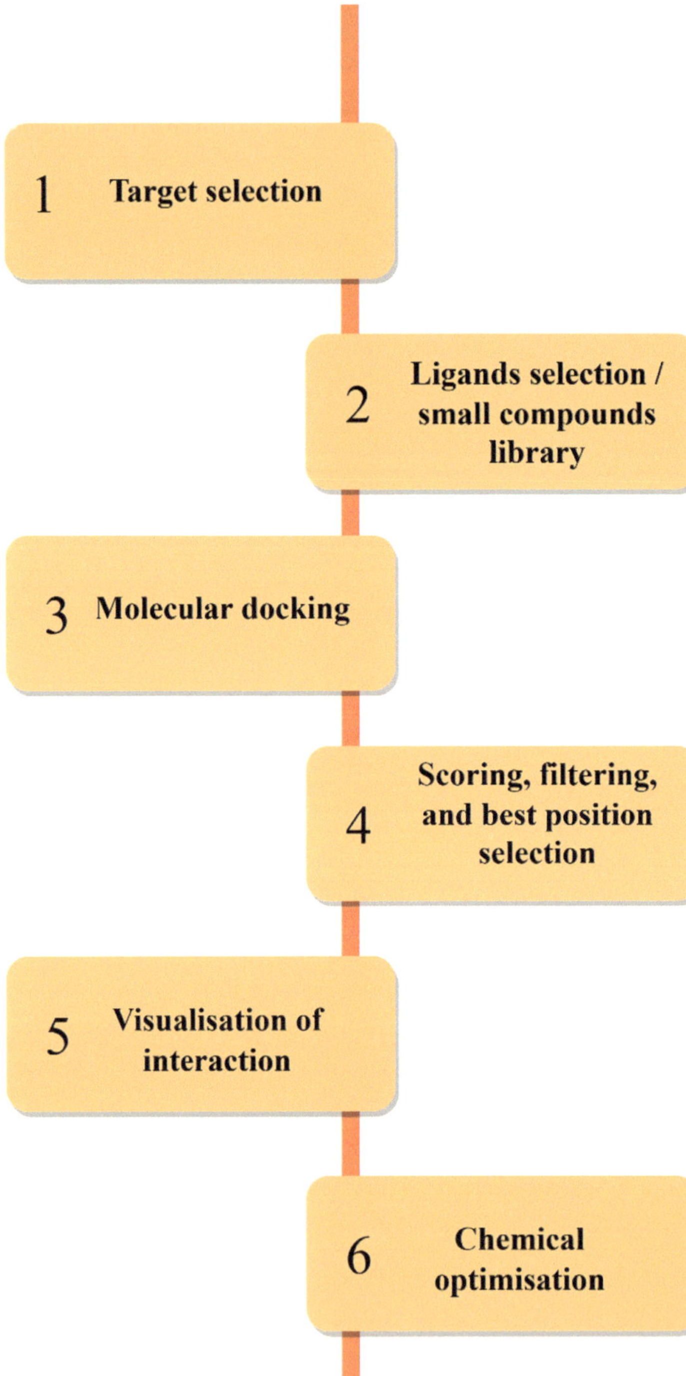

Figure 2.
Ligand-based drug design flowchart.

The resistance to monoclonal antibodies-based targeted therapy is common and rises due to the occurrence of mutations in the targeted proteins [42]. This is traced back to the heterogeneity of tumours and genomic instability.

Fortunately, a number of phytochemicals isolated from medicinal plants have been shown to decrease the capacity of tumour growth and cell proliferation, arrest the cell cycle, induce apoptosis, regulate the tumour micro-environment and inhibit metastasis and angiogenesis [43–45]. Curcumin was shown to inhibit CD44 and CD166 and metalloproteinase-2, and downregulate Gli-1, Notch-1 and cyclin D1 in various types of cancer, including colon, gastric, breast, head and neck and lung cancers. The anti-cancer activity of curcumin has been studied in silico and *in vitro* through the analysis of its capacity to specifically target EGFR, metalloproteinase-2 and NF-κB, cancer-specific proteins [46–48]. Similarly, molecular docking approach also confirmed the anticancer potential of curcumin and its analogues by showing binding interaction with the GSK-3β, EGFR and Bcr-Abl proteins. Using chemical synthesis and molecular docking, Naqvi et al. [49] have identified the inhibitory effects on oestrogen receptors of a new chemically modified bioactive curcumin. Based on the results of the computational investigation, the chemical in question is an effective oestrogen blocker due to its low binding energy and high drug-likeness ratings, where its antiproliferative effect has been proved *in vitro*. Curcumin and its derivates exert a xanthine oxidase inhibitory effect according to the in-silico study conducted by Malik et al. [50]. Using molecular docking analysis and molecular dynamic simulation, Rasul et al. [51] suggested a further lead optimisation of eugenol and its derivatives as effective anti-cancer therapeutics against breast cancer. The compounds have shown potent inhibitory effects on oestrogen receptors, progesterone receptors, EGFR, CDK2, mTOR, ERBB2, c-Src, HSP90 and chemokines receptors, breast cancer-related proteins. The compounds have displayed drug-likeness properties and stable protein-ligand complexes.

Pharmacophore-oriented molecular design using natural templates is the last resort for natural lead optimisation and helps accelerate optimisation of natural product core structures to enhance their anti-tumour activities [52–54].

3. Network pharmacology

When applied to the study of medications, targets and disorders, network analysis, systems biology and pharmacology all come together to form the developing area of network pharmacology [55]. Potential therapeutic targets can be found, drug efficacy can be predicted, drug mechanisms of action can be understood and drug repurposing can be investigated when network pharmacology is performed [56]. Drug databases, protein-protein interaction databases, gene expression data, disease-related databases and other pertinent sources of biological information are the foundation of this approach [57].

Identifying the drug's target proteins or genes is the first step [58–62]. Search for the medicines and their known targets in drug databases like DrugBank and PubChem [63–66]. Second, model the relationships among medications, targets and diseases using biological networks. Several programs and applications exist specifically for this purpose of network analysis. For instance, you can build a network that shows how drugs and diseases interact with one another [57]. Network topology analysis, cluster analysis, functional enrichment analysis and pathway analysis are all part of the analysis of the resulting network. The purpose is to discover key nodes or modules in the network that relate medications, targets and diseases [67]. The procedures of network pharmacology are depicted in **Figure 3**.

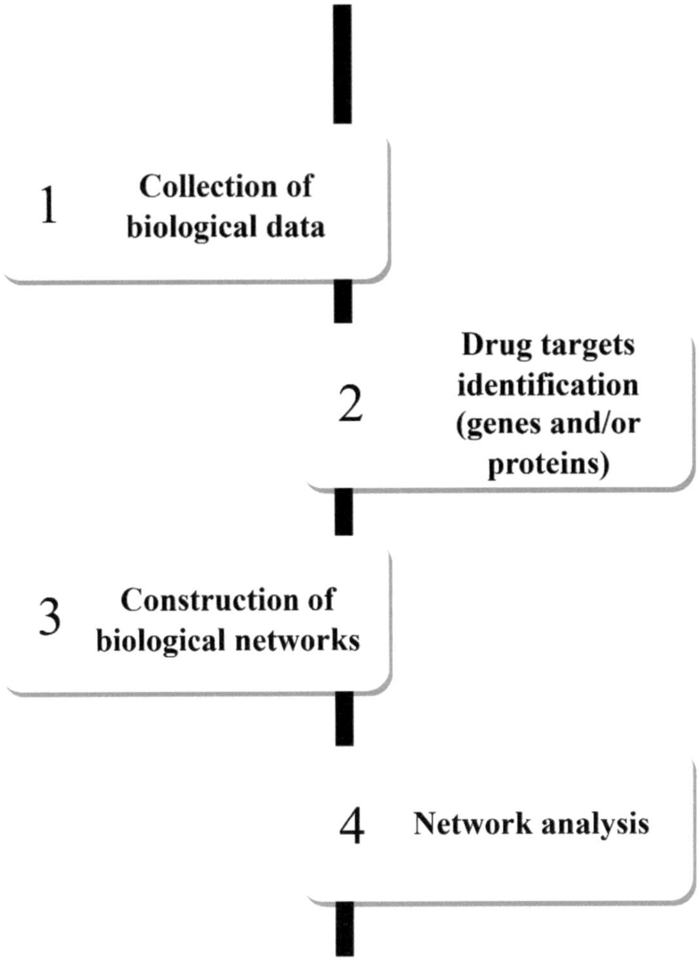

Figure 3.
Network pharmacology flowchart.

Besides Drugbank, BindingDB and Pubchem, Therapeutic Target Database (TTD) enables the identification of therapeutic targets (proteins), their functions and respective drugs [68]. In addition, Online Mendelian Inheritance in Man (OMIM) database provides information about deregulated/mutated genes implicated in various genetic diseases. Uniprot, a comprehensive protein database, provides disease-related proteins, their structure, function, variations and their involvement in diseases. Furthermore, Comparative Toxicogenomics Database (CTD) focuses on the interactions between chemicals, genes and diseases *via* the integration of data from toxicological, genomic and pharmacological aspects. Search Tool for Interactions of Chemicals (STITCH) database provides information on the chemical-protein interactions and drug-target associations. It allows the construction of interaction networks, and analyse their functional implications. Moreover, Drug Gene Interaction Database (DGIdb) and DisGeNET database provide information on the potential therapeutic implication of associated genes and drugs. They explore both drug-disease and gene-disease associations. ChEMBL database explores the interaction between bioactive compounds and the target proteins. ChEMBL provides additional information on the potency, selectivity and the binding affinity of drugs towards their disease-associated targets [69].

Regarding the network construction, various tools are available to analyse the interactions between the drug candidates, the genes and the respective diseases identified in the previous step. These tools include Cytoscape and cytoscapse.js, Search Tool for the Retrieval of Interacting Genes/Proteins (STRING), GeneMANIA, Ingenuity Pathway Analysis (IPA) and NetworkX. It is noteworthy that two types of networks exist: drug-target interaction network and drug-disease interaction network. First, drug-target interaction network represents the direct association between the identified drugs and their selected targets/proteins that they interact with [70, 71]. The molecular mechanism of the drugs on their protein/gene targets could be depicted by capturing the direct interactions between the two entities [72, 73]. However, repurposing medications, discovering new treatment opportunities and novel drug candidates and learning more about the connections between pharmaceuticals and disorders are all possible with the use of a drug-disease interaction network [74].

Different approaches can be used to explore and analyse the constructed network, including pathway analysis, functional enrichment analysis, topology analysis and clustering analysis (**Figure 4**). The topology analysis examines a network's structure and characteristics. It aids in understanding network organisation, connectivity patterns and key nodes and edges. Network topology analysis methods include the study of the network's nodes' degree distribution (number of connections of nodes) [57]. It helps detect a power-law distribution or normal distribution. Measuring the number

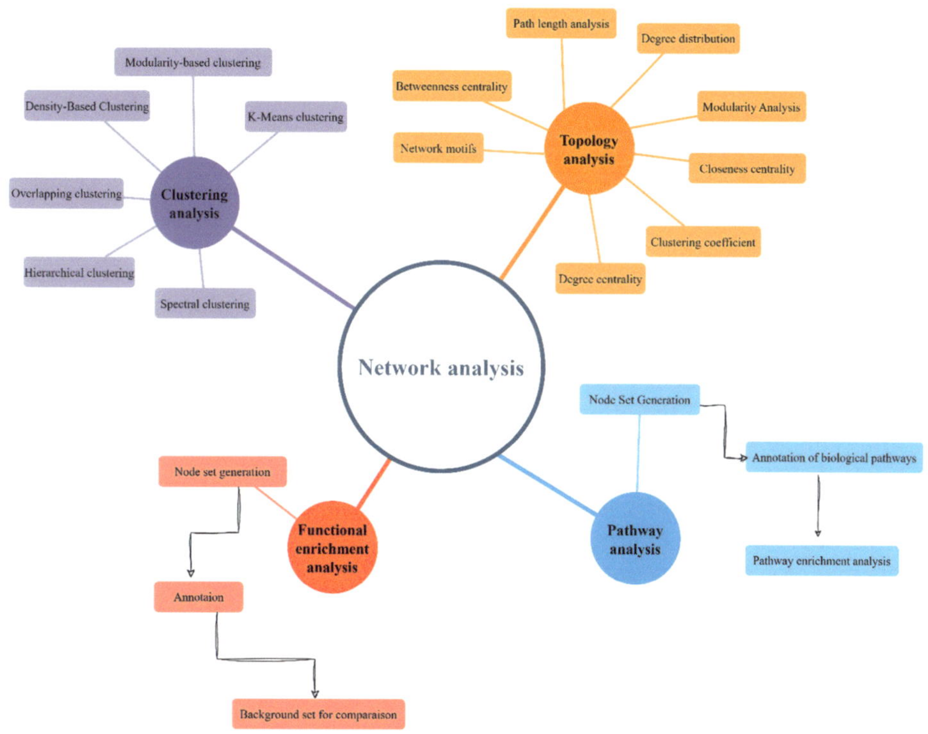

Figure 4.
Approaches used for biological network analysis.

of connections of each node presents the degree centrality analysis where central or prominent nodes have higher degrees. In addition, the betweenness centrality, how many shortest pathways a node is on, affects the interaction flow, whereas nodes with higher betweenness centrality have a greater influence on the interactions. Another topological parameter is the closeness centrality, which measures a node's network proximity. It calculates the average shortest path between nodes. High-closeness centrality nodes are more accessible and can swiftly transduce the signals in the network. The coefficient of clustering measures nodes' neighbours' connectivity, where high clustering coefficients suggest strongly connected network units. Another parameter of topology aspect is the network motifs, which are repeated interconnection patterns among a small collection of nodes revealing local connection and functional units. Moreover, modularity analysis detects coherent groups or communities of nodes in a network by comparing the density of connections between nodes in the same community to those in different communities. Finally, path length analysis finds the average shortest path between all pairs of network nodes. It shows the efficiency of signal transduction.

From another aspect, analysing the network from clustering outlook uses connection patterns to find node clusters. It seeks meaningful structural and functional network units and reveals network organisation, community structure and interactions. Common clustering analysis approaches are modularity- and density-based, hierarchical, K-Means and spectral clustering. The modularity-based clustering measures the strength of network communities (modules). It optimises the modularity score to locate groups of nodes with dense internal connections and sparse external connections. It is worth noting that the communities are located based on network structural features: the community detection method. The density-based clustering clusters dense node regions based on the density of connections within a region of the network. K-means clustering divides the network nodes into K-related clusters. In addition, overlapping clustering finds nodes that belong to numerous clusters or communities.

The analysis of a network from pathway and functional aspect aims to investigate the molecular signalling pathways that are significantly enriched among the identified genes/proteins in the constructed network. Briefly, a set of nodes is identified based on differentially expressed genes, topological features or network clusters or modules. Genes/proteins could be, then, annotated and mapped to the corresponding signalling pathways in databases like KEGG, Reactome and WikiPathways using corresponding identifiers. To annotate the nodes with relevant biological information, such as gene symbols, protein identifiers or other functional annotations, Gene Ontology (GO), KEGG and other functional databases could be used.

Interestingly, network pharmacology enable the identification of particular molecular targets and signalling pathways involved in tumorigenesis and other cancer characteristics. In addition, network pharmacology helps predict the efficacy and potential adverse effects of novel/alternative anticancer therapeutic candidates by conducting protein-protein interaction networks, drug-target networks and drug-disease networks, and by integrating gene expression data. Network pharmacology has been shown to be an effective method for investigating the breadth and depth of mechanism of action exerted by medicinal plants. Furthermore, it provides opportunity for drug repurposing in the treatment of cancer. Researchers can identify existing/novel drugs and biomolecules with the potential to modulate specific cancer-related pathways or targets. In addition, this holistic approach facilitates the identification of novel biomarkers and therapeutic targets, allows for a more comprehensive understanding of cancer biology through integration of multi-omics data and contributes to the development of precision and personalised medicine,, therefore, enhancing treatment efficacy. Potential therapeutic targets and cancer-related signalling pathways affected by drugs and plant-based chemicals can be predicted with the aid of network pharmacology. A recent study conducted by Sakle et al. [73] is one of the successful stories. The study uncovered the exact molecular mechanism of Caesalpinia pulcherima against breast cancer. The approach enabled the precise identification of four active compounds and 150 target genes involved in the anti-cancer activity of the plant. Zhang et al. [75] have been able to elucidate the potential of Rheum palmatum L. to induce apoptosis, and the exact molecular mechanism of the plant involving 16 active phytocompounds, targeting 563 lung cancer-related genes. In Lee et al. [76] have been able to elucidate the molecular mechanism exerted by three plants: Cordyceps militaris, Lonicera japonica Thunberg and Artemisia capillaris Thunberg, combined, against breast cancer. The study has demonstrated 18 phytocompounds are responsible for the anti-cancer effect by targeting 140 breast cancer-related genes. Jin et al. [77] studied the pharmacological effect of Xiao-Chai-Hu-Tang against colorectal cancer. The study revealed, precisely, the synergism of quercetin, kaempferol, stigmasterol, acacetin and baicalein to target COX-2, cyclin B1, NR3C2, CA2 and MMP1. Taken together, network pharmacology enhances the plant-based drug research, discovery and development [78].

4. Conclusion

In conclusion, because of their potential to bind and modify cellular targets implicated in cancer, natural products and medicinal plants have played a crucial role in drug discovery. Their promise in traditional medicines is highlighted by their low toxicity, low cost and convenience of availability. On the other hand, bioinformatics and databases are of vital significance to cancer research when it comes to finding therapeutic alternatives. Computer-aided drug design and network pharmacology facilitate the comprehension of drug-target interactions, the prediction of drug efficacy and adverse effects, the identification of novel drug targets and the repurposing of existing drugs. These applications enable researchers to obtain a deeper understanding of the biology of cancer and expedite the creation of effective plant-based therapeutic strategies.

Conflict of interest

The authors declare no conflict of interest.

Author details

Amel Elbasyouni[1*], Stephen Wilson Kpordze[1], Hadil Suliman Hussein[1], Oumarou Soro[1], Samuel Mulondo[2], Jonas Nshimirimana[1] and Tekeba Sisay Melese[1]

1 Department of Molecular Biology and Biotechnology, Pan African University for Basic Sciences, Technology, and Innovation (PAUSTI), Kenya

2 National Livestock Resource Research Institute, Uganda

*Address all correspondence to: elbasyouni.amel@hotmail.com

References

[1] Sung H, Ferlay J, Siegel RL, Laversanne M, Soerjomataram I, Jemal A, et al. Global cancer statistics 2020: GLOBOCAN estimates of incidence and mortality worldwide for 36 cancers in 185 countries. CA: a Cancer Journal for Clinicians. 2021;**71**(3):209-249

[2] Danaei G, Vander Hoorn S, Lopez AD, Murray CJ, Ezzati M. Causes of cancer in the world: Comparative risk assessment of nine behavioural and environmental risk factors. The Lancet. 2005;**366**(9499):1784-1793

[3] Thomas F, Roche B, Ujvari B. Intrinsic versus extrinsic cancer risks: The debate continues. Trends Cancer. 2016;**2**(2):68-69

[4] Tran KB, Lang JJ, Compton K, Xu R, Acheson AR, Henrikson HJ, et al. The global burden of cancer attributable to risk factors, 2010-19: A systematic analysis for the global burden of disease study 2019. The Lancet. 2022;**400**(10352):563-591

[5] Warnakulasuriya S. Causes of oral cancer – An appraisal of controversies. British Dental Journal. 2009;**207**(10):471-475

[6] Wu S, Zhu W, Thompson P, Hannun YA. Evaluating intrinsic and non-intrinsic cancer risk factors. Nature Communications. 2018;**9**(1):3490

[7] Wu S, Hannun Y. The importance of extrinsic factors in the development of cancers. Molecular & Cellular Oncology. 2016;**3**(3):e1143079

[8] Zhu W, Wu S, Hannun YA. Contributions of the intrinsic mutation process to cancer mutation and risk burdens. eBioMedicine. 2017;**24**:5-6

[9] Hanahan D. Hallmarks of cancer: New dimensions. Cancer Discovery. 2022;**12**(1):31-46

[10] Sever R, Brugge JS. Signal transduction in cancer. Cold Spring Harbor Perspectives in Medicine. 2015;**5**(4):a006098-a006098

[11] Abbas Z, Rehman S. An overview of cancer treatment modalities. In: Shahzad HN, editor. Neoplasm [Internet]. London: InTech; 2018 [cited 2023 May 3]. Available from: http://www.intechopen.com/books/neoplasm/an-overview-of-cancer-treatment-modalities

[12] Licciardi PV, Underwood JR. Plant-derived medicines: A novel class of immunological adjuvants. International Immunopharmacology. 2011;**11**(3):390-398

[13] Mohan L. Plant-based drugs as an adjuvant to cancer chemotherapy. In: Akram M, editor. Alternative Medicine - Update [Internet]. London, UK: IntechOpen; 2021 [cited 2023 Feb 1] Available from: https://www.intechopen.com/books/alternative-medicine-update/plant-based-drugs-as-an-adjuvant-to-cancer-chemotherapy

[14] Siddiqui AJ, Jahan S, Singh R, Saxena J, Ashraf SA, Khan A, et al. Plants in anticancer drug discovery: From molecular mechanism to chemoprevention. Kabir Y, editor. BioMed Research International. 2022;**2022**:1-18

[15] Desai A, Qazi G, Ganju R, El-Tamer M, Singh J, Saxena A, et al.

Medicinal plants and cancer chemoprevention. Current Drug Metabolism. 2008;**9**(7):581-591

[16] Cragg GM, Pezzuto JM. Natural products as a vital source for the discovery of cancer chemotherapeutic and Chemopreventive agents. Medical Principles and Practice. 2016;**25**(Suppl. 2):41-59

[17] Dehelean CA, Marcovici I, Soica C, Mioc M, Coricovac D, Iurciuc S, et al. Plant-derived anticancer compounds as new perspectives in drug discovery and alternative therapy. Molecules. 2021;**26**(4):1109

[18] Iqbal J, Abbasi BA, Mahmood T, Kanwal S, Ali B, Shah SA, et al. Plant-derived anticancer agents: A green anticancer approach. Asian Pacific Journal of Tropical Biomedicine. 2017;**7**(12):1129-1150

[19] Tuorkey MJ. Cancer therapy with phytochemicals: Present and future perspectives. Biomedical and Environmental Sciences. 2015;**28**(11):808-819

[20] Prasad V, Mailankody S. Research and Development spending to bring a single cancer drug to market and revenues after approval. JAMA Internal Medicine. 2017;**177**(11):1569

[21] Lu DY, Lu TR. Anticancer drug development, challenge and dilemma. Nursing & Care Open Access Journal. 2020;**7**(3):72-75

[22] Dangi-Garimella S. The role of bioinformatics in diabetes drug development--and precision medicine. The American Journal of Managed Care. May 2014;**20**(8 Spec No.):E1. PMID: 25617937

[23] Efferth T, Saeed MEM, Mirghani E, Alim A, Yassin Z, Saeed E, et al. Integration of phytochemicals and phytotherapy into cancer precision medicine. Oncotarget. 2017;**8**:50284-50304. Retrieved from https://www.oncotarget.com/article/17466/text/

[24] Fridlender M, Kapulnik Y, Koltai H. Plant derived substances with anti-cancer activity: From folklore to practice. Frontiers in Plant Science [Internet]. 2015 [cited 2023 May 9];**6**. Available from: http://journal.frontiersin.org/article/10.3389/fpls.2015.00799

[25] Li K, Du Y, Li L, Wei DQ. Bioinformatics approaches for anti-cancer drug discovery. Current Drug Targets. 2019;**21**(1):3-17

[26] Sharma V, Sarkar IN. Bioinformatics opportunities for identification and study of medicinal plants. Briefings in Bioinformatics. 2013;**14**(2):238-250

[27] The International Natural Product Sciences Taskforce, Atanasov AG, Zotchev SB, Dirsch VM, Supuran CT. Natural products in drug discovery: Advances and opportunities. Nature Reviews. Drug Discovery. 2021;**20**(3):200-216

[28] Batool M, Ahmad B, Choi S. A structure-based drug discovery paradigm. International Journal of Molecular Sciences. 2019;**20**(11):2783

[29] Faraggi E, Dunker AK, Sussman JL, Kloczkowski A. Comparing NMR and X-ray protein structure: Lindemann-like parameters and NMR disorder. Journal of Biomolecular Structure & Dynamics. 2018;**36**(9):2331-2341

[30] Keiffer S, Carneiro MG, Hollander J, Kobayashi M, Pogoryelev D, Ab E, et al. NMR in target driven drug discovery: Why not? Journal of Biomolecular NMR. 2020;**74**(10-11):521-529

[31] Maveyraud L, Mourey L. Protein X-ray crystallography and drug discovery. Molecules. 2020;**25**(5):1030

[32] Yee AA, Savchenko A, Ignachenko A, Lukin J, Xu X, Skarina T, et al. NMR and X-ray crystallography, complementary tools in structural proteomics of small proteins. Journal of the American Chemical Society. 2005;**127**(47):16512-16517

[33] Anderson AC. Structure-based functional Design of Drugs: From target to Lead compound. In: Espina V, Liotta LA, editors. Molecular Profiling [Internet]. Totowa, NJ: Humana Press; 2012 [cited 2023 May 21]. pp. 359-366. (Methods in Molecular Biology; Vol. 823) Available from: https://link.springer.com/10.1007/978-1-60327-216-2_23

[34] Iglesias J, Saen-oon S, Soliva R, Guallar V. Computational structure-based drug design: Predicting target flexibility. WIREs Computational Molecular Science [Internet]. 2018 Sep [cited 2023 May 21];**8**(5) Available from: https://onlinelibrary.wiley.com/doi/10.1002/wcms.1367

[35] Bajad NG, Rayala S, Gutti G, Sharma A, Singh M, Kumar A, et al. Systematic review on role of structure based drug design (SBDD) in the identification of anti-viral leads against SARS-Cov-2. Current Research in Pharmacology and Drug Discovery. 2021;**2**:100026

[36] Hardianto A, Yusuf M, Liu F, Ranganathan S. Structure-based drug design workflow. In: Encyclopedia of Bioinformatics and Computational Biology [Internet]. Elsevier; 2019 [cited 2023 May 21]. pp. 273-282 Available from: https://linkinghub.elsevier.com/retrieve/pii/B9780128096338201040

[37] Anderson AC. The process of structure-based drug design. Chemistry & Biology. 2003;**10**(9):787-797

[38] Śledź P, Caflisch A. Protein structure-based drug design: From docking to molecular dynamics. Current Opinion in Structural Biology. 2018;**48**:93-102

[39] Molla M, Aljahdali M, Sumon M, Asseri A, Altayb H, Islam M, et al. Integrative ligand-based pharmacophore Modeling, virtual screening, and molecular docking simulation approaches identified potential Lead compounds against pancreatic cancer by targeting FAK1. Pharmaceuticals. 2023;**16**(1):120

[40] Fischer A, Smieško M, Sellner M, Lill MA. Decision making in structure-based drug discovery: Visual inspection of docking results. Journal of Medicinal Chemistry. 2021;**64**(5):2489-2500

[41] Pinzi L, Rastelli G. Molecular docking: Shifting paradigms in drug discovery. International Journal of Molecular Sciences. 2019;**20**(18):4331

[42] Baudino T. Targeted cancer therapy: The next generation of cancer treatment. Current Drug Discovery Technologies. 2015;**12**(1):3-20

[43] Hosseini A, Ghorbani A. Cancer therapy with phytochemicals: evidence from clinical studies. Avicenna Journal of Phytomedicine. Mar-Apr **2015**;5(2):84-97. PMID: 25949949; PMCID: PMC4418057

[44] Sadeghnia HR, Ghorbani Hesari T, Mortazavian SM, Mousavi SH, Tayarani-Najaran Z, Ghorbani A. Viola tricolor induces apoptosis in cancer cells and exhibits antiangiogenic activity on chicken Chorioallantoic membrane. BioMed Research International. 2014;**2014**:1-8

[45] Tan W, Lu J, Huang M, Li Y, Chen M, Wu G, et al. Anti-cancer natural products isolated from chinese medicinal herbs. Chinese Medicine. 2011;**6**(1):27

[46] Praseetha NG, Divya UK, Nair S. Identifying the potential role of curcumin analogues as anti-breast cancer agents; an in silico approach. Egyptian Journal of Medical Human Genetics. 2022;**23**(1):100

[47] Saeed MEM, Yücer R, Dawood M, Hegazy MEF, Drif A, Ooko E, et al. In silico and In vitro screening of 50 curcumin compounds as EGFR and NF-κB inhibitors. International Journal of Molecular Sciences. 2022;**23**(7):3966

[48] Shefrin S, Manakadan AA, Saranya TS. A computational study of anticancer activity of curcumin derivatives using in silico drug designing and molecular docking tools. Asian Journal of Chemistry. 2018;**30**(6):1335-1339

[49] Naqvi A, Malasoni R, Gupta S, Srivastava A, Pandey R, Dwivedi A. In silico and In vitro anticancer activity of isolated novel marker compound from chemically modified bioactive fraction from Curcuma longa (NCCL). Pharmacognosy Magazine. 2017;**13**(51):640

[50] Malik N, Dhiman P, Khatkar A. In Silico Design and Synthesis of Targeted Curcumin Derivatives as Xanthine Oxidase Inhibitors. Current Drug Targets. 2019;**20**(5):593-603

[51] Rasul HO, Aziz BK, Ghafour DD, Kivrak A. In silico molecular docking and dynamic simulation of eugenol compounds against breast cancer. Journal of Molecular Modeling. 28 Dec 2021;**28**(1):17. DOI: 10.1007/s00894-021-05010-w. Erratum in: Journal of Molecular Modeling. 2022 Mar 5;28(4):78. PMID: 34962586

[52] Wu S, Ding M, Wang X, Li W, Zhao Y. 25-Methoxyl-Dammarane-3β, 12β, 20-Triol, a ginseng Saponin derivative and an anticancer agent: In vitro and In vivo activities, molecular mechanism of action, pharmacokinetics and structural modification. Medicinal Chemistry [Internet]. 2017 [cited 2023 May 21];**07**(03) Available from: https://www.omicsonline.org/open-access/25methoxyldammarane3-12-20triol-a-ginseng-saponinderivative-and-an-anticancer-agent-in-vitro-and-in-vivo-activitiesmolecular-mecha-21-61-0444-1000437.php?aid=87824

[53] Xiao Z, Morris-Natschke SL, Lee KH. Strategies for the optimization of natural leads to anticancer drugs or drug candidates: Strategies for the optimization of natural leads. Medicinal Research Reviews. 2016;**36**(1):32-91

[54] Xu Z, Eichler B, Klausner EA, Duffy-Matzner J, Zheng W. Lead/drug discovery from natural resources. Molecules. 2022;**27**(23):8280

[55] Zheng S, Xue T, Wang B, Guo H, Liu Q. Application of network pharmacology in the study of the mechanism of action of traditional chinese medicine in the treatment of COVID-19. Frontiers in Pharmacology. 2022;**13**:926901

[56] Zhou Z, Chen B, Chen S, Lin M, Chen Y, Jin S, et al. Applications of network pharmacology in traditional Chinese medicine research. Evidence-based Complementary and Alternative Medicine. 2020;**2020**:1-7

[57] Luo T, ting, Lu Y, Yan S kai, Xiao X, Rong X lu, Guo J. Network pharmacology in research of Chinese medicine formula: Methodology, application

and prospective. Chinese Journal of Integrative Medicine. 2020;**26**(1): 72-80

[58] Alegría-Arcos M, Barbosa T, Sepúlveda F, Combariza G, González J, Gil C, et al. Network pharmacology reveals multitarget mechanism of action of drugs to be repurposed for COVID-19. Frontiers in Pharmacology. 2022;**13**:952192

[59] Chen S, Jiang H, Cao Y, Wang Y, Hu Z, Zhu Z, et al. Drug target identification using network analysis: Taking active components in Sini decoction as an example. Scientific Reports. 2016;**6**(1):24245

[60] Feng Y, Wang Q, Wang T. Drug target protein-protein interaction networks: A systematic perspective. BioMed Research International. 2017;**2017**:1-13

[61] Zhao S, Iyengar R. Systems pharmacology: Network analysis to identify multiscale mechanisms of drug action. Annual Review of Pharmacology and Toxicology. 2012;**52**(1):505-521

[62] Zhao S, Li S. Network-based relating pharmacological and genomic spaces for drug target identification. PLoS One; 2010;5(7):e11764

[63] Li Q, Cheng T, Wang Y, Bryant SH. PubChem as a public resource for drug discovery. Drug Discovery Today. 2010;**15**(23-24):1052-1057

[64] Lomenick B, Olsen RW, Huang J. Identification of direct protein targets of small molecules. ACS Chemical Biology. 2011;**6**(1):34-46

[65] Schenone M, Dančík V, Wagner BK, Clemons PA. Target identification and mechanism of action in chemical biology and drug discovery. Nature Chemical Biology. 2013;**9**(4):232-240

[66] Wishart DS. DrugBank: A comprehensive resource for in silico drug discovery and exploration. Nucleic Acids Research. 2006;**34**(90001):D668-D672

[67] Kibble M, Saarinen N, Tang J, Wennerberg K, Mäkelä S, Aittokallio T. Network pharmacology applications to map the unexplored target space and therapeutic potential of natural products. Natural Product Reports. 2015;**32**(8):1249-1266

[68] Wang Y, Zhang S, Li F, Zhou Y, Zhang Y, Wang Z, et al. Therapeutic target database 2020: Enriched resource for facilitating research and early development of targeted therapeutics. Nucleic Acids Research. 2019;**48**:D1031-D1041

[69] Zhang R, Zhu X, Bai H, Ning K. Network pharmacology databases for traditional Chinese medicine: Review and assessment. Frontiers in Pharmacology. 2019;**10**:123

[70] Li L, Lu Y, Liu Y, Wang D, Duan L, Cheng S, et al. Network pharmacology analysis of Huangqi Jianzhong Tang targets in gastric cancer. Frontiers in Pharmacology. 2022;**13**:882147

[71] Wang L, Wang P, Chen Y, Li C, Wang X, Li M, et al. To explore the network pharmacology and molecular docking mechanism of Chaihu Shugan powder with the "same treatment for different diseases" for insomnia and depression based on the COVID-19 pandemic [internet]. In Review. 2022 [cited 2023 May 23]. Available from: https://www.researchsquare.com/article/rs-1332355/v2

[72] Lv L, Huang X, Li X, Fang R, Wang X, Zhong K, et al. Study on the anti-inflammatory mechanism of volatile oil of Amydrium sinense based on

network pharmacology. Journal of Physics Conference Series. 2020;**1549**(3):032024

[73] Sakle NS, More SA, Mokale SN. A network pharmacology-based approach to explore potential targets of Caesalpinia pulcherima: An updated prototype in drug discovery. Scientific Reports. 2020;**10**(1):17217

[74] Batool S, Javed MR, Aslam S, Noor F, Javed HMF, Seemab R, et al. Network pharmacology and bioinformatics approach reveals the multi-target pharmacological mechanism of Fumaria indica in the treatment of liver cancer. Pharmaceuticals. 2022;**15**(6):654

[75] Zhang Q, Liu J, Li R, Zhao R, Zhang M, Wei S, et al. A network pharmacology approach to investigate the anticancer mechanism and potential active ingredients of Rheum palmatum L against lung cancer via induction of apoptosis. Frontiers in Pharmacology. 2020;**11**:528308

[76] Lee HS, Lee IH, Kang K, Park SI, Moon SJ, Lee CH, et al. A network pharmacology study on the molecular mechanisms of FDY003 for breast cancer treatment. Evidence-based Complementary and Alternative Medicine : eCAM. 2021;**2021**:1-18

[77] Jin J, Chen B, Zhan X, Zhou Z, Liu H, Dong Y. Network pharmacology and molecular docking study on the mechanism of colorectal cancer treatment using Xiao-chai-Hu-Tang. PLoS One. 2021;**16**(6):e0252508

[78] Lin L, Chen W, Yao C, Wu L, Yan Q, Cai X, et al. Exploring the target and molecular mechanism of Astragalus membranaceus in the treatment of vascular cognitive impairment based on network pharmacology and molecular docking. Medicine (Baltimore). 2023;**102**(12):e33063

Chapter 3

Spices Are Also Medicine: Some Studies on Antioxidant and Antibacterial Activities of Spice Plants in Vietnam

Le Quynh Mai

Abstract

Spices are commonly used in the daily meals of Vietnamese families. They not only bring a specific flavor to the dishes but are also drugs that help naturally increase disease resistance. Spices are also used in folk remedies to cure or prevent certain diseases. When the world faces the quick change of pathogenic microorganisms, antibiotic-resistant bacteria regularly appear, then searching for more natural sources of medicine becomes necessary. Many studies have been conducted to screen bioactive substances from the rich and diverse plant sources of Vietnam. Extracts from spices and several spice mixtures were evaluated for their antioxidant and antimicrobial activities, indicating their potential as medicine. In this chapter, some research on the antioxidant and antibacterial activities of spice plants in Vietnam and some traditional ways to use spices as medicine will be presented.

Keywords: antibacterial activity, antioxidant activity, folk remedy, medicinal plant, spice plant, traditional therapy

1. Introduction

Plant-based spices are added to dishes to give them a certain smell and taste. In the cuisine arts of countries around the world, the combination of spices helps to create the characteristics of each dish as well as the characteristics of each country's cuisine. Although spices and herbs are often classified as spices which are the dry parts of the plant and herbs as the leaves [1], Vietnamese people often use both fresh and dry types as spices.

Vietnamese food culture is diverse with many delicious dishes. The spices are associated with the dish's main ingredients such as galangal with dog meat, lime leaves with chicken, ginger with fish, lemongrass with shrimp. The spices are also associated with the cooking methods, for example, garlic with stir-fried dishes, lime or kumquat with salads, ginger or lemongrass with boiled dishes, five-spice powder (mixture of cinnamon, fennel seeds, star anise, Sichuan peppercorn, and cloves) with fried or grinned dishes. Spices are essential ingredients to create the characteristics

IntechOpen

of Vietnamese dishes, and they are commonly used in the daily life of Vietnamese families. Spices are also used as natural drugs in folk remedies to cure or prevent certain diseases.

Many studies in the world have been conducted with spices [2–11]. The antibacterial activity of six common spices including clove (*Syzygium aromaticum* L.), black pepper (*Piper nigrum* L.), turmeric (*Curcuma longa* Linn), ajowan (*Trachyspermum ammi* L.), coriander (*Coriandrum sativum* L.), and cinnamon (*Cinnamomum zeylanicum* Bl.) against 10 bacteria strains was studied. The results indicated that the main active compounds in those spices were probably in their essential oils and cinnamon followed by clove had the highest antibacterial capacity [2]. An elaborate review that consulted 241 pieces of literature on antibacterial and antifungal characteristics in spices was also performed. Thereby that summarized the evaluating studies about the antibacterial ability of spices such as cinnamon, black pepper, coriander, clove (*Eugenia caryophyllata*), oregano (*Origanum vulgare*), thyme (*Thymus vulgaris*), cumin (*Cuminum cyminum*), rosemary (*Rosmarinus officinalis*), garlic (*Allium sativum*), ginger (*Zingiber officinale*), basil (*Ocimum basilicum*), fennel (*Foeniculum vulgare*), and galangal (*Alpinia galangal*). Many other spices were also determined by anti-microorganisms such as yarrow, cardamon, dill, calamint, croton, poejo, hyssop, lavender, lichen, nutmeg, basil, aniseed, savory [3].

The diversity of plants that can be used as spices is enormous. Beside popular spices that are mentioned previously, there are many others such as rosy garlic, wild garlic, oriental mustard, black cumin, chili pepper, bitter orange, common croton, horned poppy, common fennel, bay laurel, fever tea, mountain pepper, lemon balm, peppermint, myrtle, lesser cat-mint, black cumin, holy basil or tulsi, clove basil, common olive, sweet marjoram, African long pepper or wild pepper, Sicilian sumac or elm-leaved sumac, garden sage, campion, summer savory, black thyme or Mediterranean thyme [3]. There are some problems in identifying them. Many spices are commonly named after regions; however, it is not clear the region of plant growth or the place where the spices are used. For example, Ethiopian cardamom, Persian shallot, Indonesian cinnamon, Persian cumin, Mexican oregano, Spartan oregano, English mint, Macassar nutmeg, Dutch myrtle, American basil, African basil, Java tea, Syrian rue, Jerusalem sage, Mediterranean thyme, Sicilian sumac, Jamaica pepper, African long pepper, Ashanti pepper or Benin pepper. There are many synonymous scientific names for the same spices; for example, *Trachyspermum ammi* and *Carum capticum* (ajwain or ajowan), *Eugenia caryophyllata* and *Syzygium aromaticum* (clove). Some relative species belong to the same genus but are called with different common names as different spices, for example, small peppermint (*Thymus piperella*) and creeping thyme (*Thymus serpyllum*). Even, one certain plant species is called as different spices, for example, conehead thyme or Persian-hyssop, or Spanish oregano all are *Thymus capitata* (or *Thymus capitatus*). Some plants are used without any common name such as *Thymus eigii*.

Spices are known to have many antioxidants [4–6, 11]. They are mainly bioactive secondary metabolites of plants, which consist of terpenes, phenolic compounds, and nitrogen-containing compounds. The mechanisms such as blocking free radicals, acting as oxygen scavengers, and chelating metal ions capable of catalyzing oxidation are the main actions of antioxidants [4]. The antioxidant capacity of spices has been assessed mainly because of their essential oils, so fresh herbs are often found to have high antioxidant capacity. Therefore, the extraction solvent affects the antioxidant capacity of spices in the studies [4, 6]. Daily, spices are often used raw, in hot water, or soaking in wine for a period (then using wine). Water and alcohol solvents become important solvents when evaluating the effectiveness of spices as natural antioxidants. Milda E. Embuscado reviewed the antioxidant activity of hot water extracts of spices and showed four spices including clove, thyme, rosemary, and savory that had DPPH radical scavenging activities higher than 50% [4]. Usually, spices are used in combination rather than individually, so studies on the differences in bioactivities of individual spices and the combination of spices and mixtures of spices with some other compounds are also of interest [5].

In Vietnam, studies on the antibacterial and antioxidant activities of spices have also been conducted on a wide range of species, varieties, cultured areas, methods of extracting bioactive compounds, etc. In this chapter, several studies are mentioned as examples of the priority research directions on spices in Vietnam. More importantly, some traditional therapies of using spices in disease prevention and treatment are presented for readers to understand more about the role of spices in Vietnam.

2. Some research on the antioxidant and antibacterial activities of spices in Vietnam

In Vietnam, through traditional uses, there have been some summaries on the antibacterial and antioxidant capacities of daily used spices [12, 13]. Many spices are also mentioned in the list of medicinal plants in Vietnam [13, 14]. Since 1961, the direct extracts from garlic (*Allium sativum* L.) and fragrant garlic (*Allium odorum* L.) in Vietnam have been found that have antibacterial activity against seven bacteria strains (according to [13]). Inhibition zone diameters of the fresh garlic extract were greater from 1.5 to 2.5 times than fragrant garlic extract, and they lost their activities if used in the form of decoction. Vietnamese balm (*Elsholtzia ciliata*) is known as effective in treating many diseases, including flu, cold, allergies, bleeding nose, and ban on speech (traditional ion therapy also mentions leprosy). A study on Vietnamese balm showed that its essential oil contains many active substances and the most abundant was verbenol. Vietnamese balm essential oil inhibited the growth of *E. coli* as well as *Salmonella* [15].

Searching for new effective and safe cures, and new therapeutic modalities in disease prevention and treatment has always been of great interest to researchers in the world. In recent years, studies on bioactivities and bioactivity compounds from plants have also been widely conducted in Vietnam. And beside medicinal plants, spices are a group of plants that are of great interest. In studies on antibacterial activity, spices were studied and compared with medicinal plants [16]. According to the research on *in vitro* antibacterial activity of 18 eligible herbs and 21 medicinal plants against six strains of *Burkholderia pseudomallei* (causative agent of melioidosis), and seven other enteric bacteria, garlic, and fragrant garlic juices showed a broad spectrum of antimicrobial activity but lost its activity when was treated with high temperature [16]. The juice, the aqueous extract, and the alcohol extract of different plant parts were also tested and compared quite often because of the traditional ways to use the spices. The bioactivity compounds of plants may vary in content in different parts of plants grown in different regions [17, 18]. Lemongrass (*Cymbopogon citratus*) plants from three provinces: Hoa Binh, Ha Nam, and Nam Dinh were separately extracted essential oil in stems and leaves [18]. The results showed that lemongrass essential oil had antibacterial activities against *Enterococcus faecalis*, *Shigella flexneri*, *Escherichia coli*, *Streptococcus pneumoniae*, *Staphylococcus aureus*, and *Klebsiella pneumoniae* but not *Salmonella typhi*. Lemongrass oil extracts from stems inhibited the growth of bacteria better than extracts from leaves. Essential oil from Hoa Binh province lemongrass has both better antioxidant and antibacterial properties than plants from other provinces. Especially, the essential oil from both leaves and stems of plants collected from Nam Dinh province did not have anti-*Streptococcus pneumoniae* activity, while those collected from the other two provinces did [18]. There are some fruits that fruit juice is commonly used to drink as lime and kumquat are considered spices in Vietnam. Kumquat (*Citrus japonica* Thumb.) is one of the decoration plants in the traditional Tet holiday in Vietnam as the symbol of prosperity and affluence. In folk remedies, kumquat can be used as an ingredient for cough treatment and digestive support, and is good for the liver and spleen. Biological active substances contain in lime (*Citrus aurantifolia*) juice can reduce scurvy, a vitamin C deficiency symptom that leads to gingivitis, spontaneous bleeding, and weakness. Lime is used to treat fever and cough, and indigestion in tradition. Recently, studies have shown that lime concentrate has antibacterial and antioxidant properties and has a protective function against liver cell damage due to the harmful effects of alcohol (following the review in [19]). The combination of lemongrass stalks and the peels of lime, ginger tubers, and kumquat peels were tested for antioxidant and antibacterial activities and comparison of their activities with the activities of some medical plants was made [20]. The extract of ginger and kumquat mixture at the concentration of 0.1 mg/ml presented the highest free radical scavenging activity in the study. The activity even was 1.4 to 1.6 times greater than *Pluchea indica* and *Stephania glabra* (two medicinal plants). Extract of ginger and kumquat mixture was also effective in inhibition against *Bacillus cereus*, *Staphylococcus aureus*, and *Vibrio parahaemolyticus* through the agar well diffusion assay greater than *Drynaria fortunei* and P. *indica*; however, less than the ability of the extract of *S. glabra* [20]. The antibacterial ability of spices in addition to drug development applications for humans has also been studied with pathogenic micro-organisms on animals and plants applied in the fields of agriculture, cultivation, and animal husbandry [21, 22].

The comparison between the antioxidant abilities of close species or different varieties was done in Vietnam due to the enormous diversity of plants. Antiseptic, deworming, and detoxification of vines in family of *Paederia* attract the attention of researchers. A study that assessed and compared the antioxidant activity of sewer vines (*P. lanuginose* Wall.) and stink vines (*P. foetida* L.) was done [23]. Vine leaves are found to have high levels of polyphenols and vitamin C, which mainly contribute to the antioxidant activity of their extracts. The drying process may cause the decrease in bioactivity [23]. Ethanol extracts of three spices: turmeric (*Curcuma longa*), green turmeric (*C. yunnanensis*), lesser alpinia (*Alpinia conchigera*), and five other plants were tested antioxidant and antifungal activities in a study [24]. The total polyphenol content in *C. longa* extract was about 4.5 times higher than in *C. yunnanensis* (44,87 ± 0,14 compared to 10,07 ± 0,18 mg GAE/g extract), while the flavonoid content of green turmeric was light higher (144,98 and 110,75 ± 6,38 mg QE/g extract). *A. conchigera* was observed possessing highest flavonoid content in ethanol extract, 2.5 times higher than turmeric. Research has also shown that turmeric (yellow turmeric) has a higher antioxidant capacity than green turmeric [24]. It is understandable why yellow turmeric is used more commonly than green turmeric.

Other research directions with spices (as well as with bioactive plants) are the study of methods to evaluate extract composition, protocols to extract, and purify of potential bioactive compounds beside evaluating bioactive activities [25, 26]. The development of nanotechnology with the potential of targeted drug delivery is also a new research direction using extracts from spices. Turmeric became a potential object of nano-research due to its well-known active ingredient curcumin [27–29]. Then, other spices have also been noticed. Some bioactive compounds found in spices as rutin, allicin, gallic acid, quercetin, ... are the potential materials for nanoparticle formation. A study was done to synthesize silver nanoparticles using shallot (*Allium ascalonicum* L.) in Nong Lam University, Ho Chi Minh City. Pleasant Himalayan mint (*Elsholtizia blanda*) and Padang cassia (*Cinnamomum burmanni*) were in the list of 19 plants screened for synthesis silver nanoparticles in the University of Medicine and Pharmacy in Hanoi [14]. The bioactivity of nano-spices was also tested. Nano-silver particles synthesized using ginger extract as a reducing agent have shown antibacterial activity on both Gram (−) and Gram (+) strains presentative by *E. coli* and *S. aureus* [30].

3. Some traditional ways to use spices as medicine in Vietnam

In Vietnam traditional methods to prevent flu raw garlic, ginger, galangal, lemongrass, as well as scallion are regularly used. In the countryside, many families have a bottle of alcohol at home with soaked garlic inside, to cure the flu, fever, back pain, stomach pain, difficult digestion, flatulence, running nose, stuffy nose or even sinusitis, and hypertension. Parts of plants such as leaves, bud, flower, fruit, seeds, root, rhizome, stem or even bark are used as spices, as well as medicine. There are many ways to make spices into medicine. Eating raw spices is easy and common and can be daily used but to treat certain diseases the dose needs to be increased. Fresh juice of

Scientific name	Vietnamese name/ common name	Treatment diseases	Ways to use
Allium fistulosum L.	Hành/ spring onion, scallion	Cough, expectorant, diuretic, reduce malaria, edema	Eat raw Drink scallion juice
		Blister	Apply crushed leaves to the pain
		Pustules	Scallion essential oil
		Rhinitis, stuffy nose	Drop scallion juice into the nostrils
		Threatened miscarriage	Decoction
Allium odorum L. or *A. tuberosum* Roxb.	Hẹ/ fragrant garlic	Cough, diarrhea, flu, flatulence	Eat raw Drink fresh juice
		Nocturnal emission	Aqueous extracts of leaves or fruits
Allium sativum L.	Tỏi/garlic	Flu, typhoid, cholera, diphtheria	Eat raw or drink garlic juice
		Dysentery	Garlic crushed in water, filter to extract garlic water to drink and apply to the pain
		Flu, sinusitis, bronchitis hypertension	Garlic wine
		Snake bite	Apply crushed garlic to the pain

Scientific name	Vietnamese name/ common name	Treatment diseases	Ways to use
Alpinia officinarum Hance	Riềng/ galangal	Stomachache, diarrhea, flatulence, indigestion, cold, fever, vomiting	Decoction Drink fresh juice Galangal wine
		Toothache	Chew raw galangal
Amomum aromaticum Roxb.	Thảo quả/cardamon	Malaria, stomachache, vomiting, phlegm, poor spleen function	Use fruit powder
		Halitosis	Crush fruits, keep in mouth
Amomum longiligulare and *A. villosum* Lour., *Acanthospermum xanthioides* Wall.	Sa nhân/ amomum	Toothache	Keep seeds in mouth
		Stomachache, flatulence, indigestion, cholera, dysentery	Eat seeds
Anethum graveolens L. or *Peucedanum graveolens*	Thìa là/dill	Cold stomach, flatulence, vomiting, urinary retention	decoction of dried plant
		Mother's milk insufficiency	Essential oil extract from fruits
Cinnamomum loureirii Nees. and *Cinnamomum cassia, C. zeylanicum*	Quế/cinnamon	Arm and leg spasms/ cramps, Back and knee numbness, abdominal pain, menstrual blockage/ amenorrhea, urinary retention	Cinnamon powder Cinnamon tea
Coleus aromaticus Benth or *C. crassifolius* Benth	Húng chanh/ soup-mint	Flu, cough, asthma,	Eat raw Drink fresh juice
		Insect stings	Apply crushed leaves to the pain
Coriandrum sativum L.	Mùi/coriander	Reduce complications of measles	Apply crushed coriander fruits mix with coriander wine to the body
		Cold, cough, fever, headache	Aqueous coriander
		Mother's milk insufficiency	Boil coriander fruits in water, drink the water twice a day
Curcuma longa L. or *C. domestica* Lour. And *C. xanthorrhiza*	Nghệ/turmeric	Wound, get a burn	Apply fresh rhizome extraction to the pain
		Stomach ulcers	Eat turmeric powder/ turmeric powder mix with honey
		Hemoptysis, nosebleed	Orally use turmeric powder with water
		Skin swelling, arthritis	Turmeric wine
		Infected wound, uterine ulcer, cervicitis	Turmeric oil

Scientific name	Vietnamese name/ common name	Treatment diseases	Ways to use
Cymbopogon nardus Rendl and *Cymbopogon citratus*	Sả/ citronella grass and lemon grass	Urinary retention, fever	Drink fresh juice from stack or decoction Lemongrass essential oil
Elsholtzia cristata Willd or *E. ciliata* (Thunb.) Hyl.	Kinh giới/ Vietnamese balm or crested late summer mint	Fever, headache, nosebleeds, bloody stools, bloody urine	Decoction (dried whole plant)
		Loss speech	Make tea with dried flower powder
		Allergies	
Enhydra fluctuans Lour. or *Cryphiospermum repens*, *Hingtsha repens*, *Tetraotis paludosa*	Ngổ/helencha, water cress, buffalo spinach	Abdominal distension, hemorrhage, hemoptysis	Decoction (shoots)
		Inflammation	Apply crushed shoots
Houttuynia cordata Thumb.	Diếp cá/ fish mint	Hemorrhoids, pimples	Eat raw Drink fresh juice Apply crushed leaves to the pain
		Headache	Apply crushed leaves on forehead
		Irregular menstruation, urinary retention	Decoction (dried whole plant)
Illicium verum Hook.f.	Hồi/star anise	Indigestion	Decoction (fruits)
		Pain, numbness	Apply star anise wine to the pain
Mentha arvensis L.	Cây bạc hà/ corn mint	Flu, cough, stuffy nose,	Eat raw Drink fresh juice
		Headache	Massage forehead with mint oil
		Rash	Apply crushed leaves
Ocimum basilicum L.	Húng quế/basil	Sore throat, chicken cough, stomachache, toothache	Eat raw leaves Use essential oil
		Constipation, urinary retention,	Aqueous extract
Paederia tomentosa L. or *P. foetida*	Mơ tam thể/ skunkvine	Dysentery	Eat fried egg mixed with small cut leaves
		Kidney stones, urinary retention	Decoction leaves
		Rheumatism and numbness	Drink juice extracted from leaves and massage with residue
Perilla frutescens	Tía tô/ Vietnamese perilla	Cough, digestive stimulant, pain relief, detoxification	Eat raw or dried leaves
		Asthma, rheumatism	Decoction dried fruits

Scientific name	Vietnamese name/ common name	Treatment diseases	Ways to use
Petroselinum sativum Hoff. or *Carum petroselium*	Mùi tây/Persil	Urinary retention, irregular menstruation	Decoction fruits
		Inflammation	Apply crushed leaves
Piper lolot C. De	Lá lốt/lolot	Bone pain, rheumatism,	Decoction dried leaves
		Diarrhea	Decoction dried leaves
		Sweaty feet/hands	Foot/hand bath with warm water of slowly cook dried leaves
Piper nigrum L.	Tiêu/black pepper	Stomachache, cold	Pepper wine
		Indigestion	Pepper/ pepper powder
Polygonum odoratum Lour.	Răm/ Vietnamese coriander	Reduce libido, vomiting, urinary retention	Eat raw
		Ringworm, impetigo	Crush leaves, add wine and apply to the pain
		Snake bite	Crush leaves, extract juice to drink, and apply residue to the pain
Syzygium aromaticum L. or *Eugenia caryophyllata*	Đinh hương/clove	Diarrhea, vomiting, stomachache, indigestion	Use dried clove buds
		Toothache	Clove essential oil
Zingiber officinalle Rose	Gừng/ginger	Vomiting	Take a slice of ginger
		Sore throat, cough	Drink hot water/tea adding ginger Take a slice of candied ginger
		Cold, flu, headache	Massage body with ginger wine
		Cholera, dysentery	Grind dried ginger, orally use with rice water or porridge

Table 1.
Vietnamese traditional ways to use spices to treat common diseases [12, 13].

spices that are extracted by grinding or crushing fresh material and extract solution. The same way to make fresh juice but in addition of an amount of water can be done with fresh and dried spices after filtering aqueous extracts are obtained. Spice of wine is obtained by soaked materials in water or in wine (alcohol) in a period. Decoction means slowly cooking/boiling the plant parts in water. With wounds, skin diseases or diseases of muscles, bones and joints, spices can be crushed or chopped and applied to the painful area. Sometime spices are pulverized into fine powders, and sometimes spices tea can be made by being kept in hot water for a while. Essential oils are quite often extracted from both fresh and dried spices depending on the species. The ways to use individual spices were summarized (**Table 1**).

Spices are also used in combination with each other and with some other herbs or plants to treat several diseases in daily life (**Table 2**).

Combination	Disease treatment	Way to use
Dried ginger, galangal	Malaria, fever, loss of appetite	Mix grind powders with pig gallbladder fluid to make pills, orally use the pills
Ginger, cardamon, chebulic myrobalan - kha tử (*Terminalia chebula* Retz.)	Malaria, a cold, dehydration, loss of appetite	Decoction
Dried ginger, licorice—cam thảo (*Glycyrrhiza glabra*)	Headache, cold stomach, vomiting, phlegm	Decoction
Ginger, rhizome of Bengal arum—bán hạ chế (*Typhonium trilobatum* (L.) Schott.)	Asthma, vomiting	Decoction
Black pepper, Bengal arum, ginger	Diarrhea and vomiting	Equal mixture of grinded pepper and Bengal arum, orally use with ginger water
Dried fish mint, common jujube—táo tàu (*Ziziphus jujuba*) fruit	Middle ear swelling, milk duct swelling	Decoction
Galangal, lemon grass, pomelo—bưởi (*Citrus maxima* (Burm.) Merr.)	Flu, cold	Boil leaves in water, take a bath
Vietnamese perilla, lemon grass, bamboo—tre (*Bambusa arundinacea* (Retz.) Willd.), pomelo	Flu, cold	Boil leaves in water, take a bath
Vietnamese balm, Vietnamese perilla, tulsi—hương nhu (*Ocimum sanctum* L.)	Vomiting	Eat raw mixture of leaves
Vietnamese balm, ginger	Arthritis	Apply crushed leaves adding with crushed ginger to the pain

Table 2.
Some of the spices combination and spices combine with other plants are used in disease treatment [13].

4. Conclusion

Plant-based spices are used in daily life to help us naturally resist some common diseases. We can still rely on spices to be cured from runny nose, headache, cold, and flu without knowing it. It is thanks to the antibacterial and antioxidant properties of spices that they can resist diseases. Spices also have antifungal activity, the ability to inhibit cancer cell development, increase resistance, immune system support, supplement nutrition, etc. Spices have been and will be a potential source for research and development of new drugs. Indeed, spices have long been present in Vietnamese remedies to treat several diseases as summarized in this chapter. Research on spices will still be carried out more deeply and widely to exploit this marvelous source of medicine.

Author details

Le Quynh Mai
University of Science, Vietnam National University, Hanoi, Vietnam

*Address all correspondence to: lequynhmai80@vnu.edu.vn

References

[1] Shabir, Ahmad RIM, Kamran Khan M, Haseeb Ahmad M, Sajid Arshad M, Ateeq H, et al. Introductory chapter: Herbs and spices - an overview. In: Ahmad RS, editor. Herbs and Spices - New Processing Technologies. London, UK: IntechOpen; 2021. DOI: 10.5772/intechopen.100725

[2] Dinesh M, Anjana S, Binod L, Shaila B, Lekhnath SG. Study on antibacterial activity of common spices. Nepal Journal of Science and Technology. 2011;**12**:312-317. DOI: 10.3126/njst.v12i0.6518

[3] Liu Q, Meng X, Li Y, Zhao CN, Tang GY, Li HB. Antibacterial and antifungal activities of spices. International Journal of Molecular Sciences. 2017;**18**(6):1283. DOI: 10.3390/ijms18061283

[4] Embuscado ME. Spices and herbs: Natural sources of antioxidants – A mini review. Journal of Functional Foods. 2015;**18**:811-819. DOI: 10.1016/j.jff.2015.03.005

[5] Hossain MB, Ahmed L, Martin-Diana AB, Brunton NP, Barry-Ryan C. Individual and combined antioxidant activity of spices and spice Phenolics. Antioxidants (Basel). 2023;**12**(2):308. DOI: 10.3390/antiox12020308

[6] Yashin A, Yashin Y, Xia X, Nemzer B. Antioxidant activity of spices and their impact on human health: A review. Antioxidants. 2017;**6**(3):70. DOI: 10.3390/antiox6030070

[7] Khatri P, Rani A, Hameed S, Chandra S, Chang CM, Pandey RP. Current understanding of the molecular basis of spices for the development of potential antimicrobial medicine. Antibiotics (Basel). 2023;**12**(2):270. DOI: 10.3390/antibiotics12020270

[8] George J, Edwards D, Pun S, Williams D. Evaluation of antioxidant capacity (ABTS and CUPRAC) and Total phenolic content (Folin-Ciocalteu) assays of selected fruit, vegetables, and spices. International Journal of Food Science. 2022;**2022**:2581470. DOI: 10.1155/2022/2581470

[9] Duarte NBA, Takahashi JA. Plant spices as a source of antimicrobial synergic molecules to treat bacterial and viral Co-infections. Molecules. 2022;**27**(23):8210. DOI: 10.3390/molecules27238210

[10] Madonna Ngwatshipane Mashabela PTNaWOM. Herbs and spices' antimicrobial properties and possible use in the food sector. In: Ivanišová E, editor. Herbs and Spices - New Advances. London, UK: IntechOpen; 2022. DOI: 10.5772/intechopen.108143

[11] Rubio L, Motilva MJ, Romero MP. Recent advances in biologically active compounds in herbs and spices: A review of the most effective antioxidant and anti-inflammatory active principles. Critical Reviews in Food Science and Nutrition. 2013;**53**(9):943-953. DOI: 10.1080/10408398.2011.574802

[12] Mai VQ, Le TVN, Ngo QV, Nguyen THN, Kiet T. Popular Spices Plants in Vietnam. 3rd ed. Ho Chi Minh city, Vietnam: Agriculture Publishing House; 2000

[13] Do TL. Medicinal Plants and Medicines from Plants in Vietnam. 8th ed. Hanoi, Vietnam: Medical Publishing House; 2004

[14] Trieu AD. Screening Medicinal Plant Extracts for Synthesizing Silver Nanoparticles [Thesis]. Hanoi: VNU-University of Medicine and Pharmacy; 2021

[15] Tran TQA, Vo TTH. Study on the chemical composition and antibacterial properties of Vietnamese balm essential oil (Elsholtzia ciliata) HUAF. Journal of Agricultural Science & Technology. 2022;**6**(1):2881-2890. DOI: 10.46826/huaf-jasat.v6n1y2022.649

[16] Trinh TT, Vu TA, Bui LNH, Nguyen HV, Nguyen DTH, Dang NX, et al. Thermal and gastric stability of antimicrobial activity of juices and aqueous extracts prepared from common eligible herbs and traditional medicinal plants against Burkholderia pseudomallei and other enteric bacteria. Future Journal of Pharmaceutical Sciences. 2022;**8**(1):35-50. DOI: 10.1186/s43094-022-00424-6

[17] Nguyen MH. Hydrodistillation of essential oils from rhizome of Zingiber officinale roscoe cultivated in Phu Yen and Binh Duong provinces. HCMCOUJS. 2022;**17**(2):79-88. DOI: 10.46223/HCMCOUJ.tech.vi.17.2.2187.2022

[18] Nguyen TTM, Tran BT, Do TKTT, Truong VQ, Chien T, TDL M. Determination of biological activities and antimicrobial ability of Cymbopogon citratus essential oil in Norrthern Vietnam. In: The 4th National Scientific Conference on Biological Research and Teaching in Vietnam; Proceeding of the 4th National Scientific Conference on Biological Research and Teaching in Vietnam. Hanoi, Vietnam: Vietnam Journal of Science and Technology; 2020. pp. 680-686

[19] Huynh TD, Kha CT, Nguyen TD, Nguyen SH, Vo TNM. Quality parameters of lime fruits (citrus sp.) cultivated in long an province. Can Tho University Journal of Science. 2021;**57**(Food Technology section):170-176. DOI: 10.22144/ctu.jsi.2021.019

[20] Le TA, Pham TTH, Nguyen TBL, Le QM. Initial evaluation of antioxidant and antibacterial activities of several medicinal plant extracts collected in Vietnam. VNU Journal of Science: Natural Sciences and Technology. 2021;**37**(3):1-8. DOI: 10.25073/2588-1140/vnunst.5306

[21] Tran HTN, Tran TT, Kim NT, Nguyen TN. Preliminary study on antimicrobial properties of garlic (Allium sativum L.) for the treatment of Aeromonas hydrophila disease in Thai frog (Rana tigerina). In: Proceeding of the 4th National Fisheries Science Conference for Youth. Ho Chi Minh City: Nong Lam University; 6-7 Jun 2013. pp. 482-488

[22] Tran TPD, Luu TPK, Huynh TTQ, Nguyen TTQ. Antimicrobial activity of extracts of garlic (Allium sativum) and marjoram (Elsholtzia ciliata) against Edwardsiella ictaluri causing disease in catfish (Pangasianodon hypophthalmus). HCMC-University of Education Journal of Science. 2022;**19**(9):1472-1484. DOI: 10.54607/hcmue.js.19.9.3379(2022)

[23] Nguyen TVA, Le TQN, Tran TQA, Phan DDT, Doan TTT, Nguyen VH. Study on antioxidant activities of Paederia lanuginosa Wall. extract. In: Vietnam National Conference “Research on Application of Mechanics - Technology to Meet Industry 40” in 2019. Hue, Vietnam: Hue University; 6 April 2019. pp. 195-204. DOI: 10.46826/huaf-jasat.v3n2y2019.259

[24] Dai TXT, Tran CL, Le BH, Pham KNH, Phung TH. Antifungal and antioxidant activity of some plant extracts of the family Zingiberaceae and Dioscoreaceae. Can Tho University Journal of Science. 2020;**56**(5):52-59. DOI: 10.22144/ctu.jvn.2020.111

[25] Le VC. Research on chemical composition and structural determination of some substances in the rhyzome extract of galangal (Alpinia purpurata). In: Hoi an

City - Quang Nam Province [Thesis]. Da Nang, Vietnam: Da Nang University; 2011

[26] Nguyen TYP, Huynh NDB. Study on green extraction of antioxidants from garlic bulbs (Allium sativum L.). Can Tho University Journal of Science. 2020;**56**(1):124-135. DOI: 10.22144/ctu.jvn.2020.013

[27] Hoang LS, Nguyen THT, Do TS, Mai NTA. Effect of nanocurcumin particles prepared by top-down method on CCl4 induced hepatic fibrosis mice. International Journal of Pharmaceutical Sciences and Research. 2013;**4**(12):4542-4548. DOI: 10.13040/ijpsr.0975-8232.4(12).4542-48

[28] Le TKA, Le DV, Vo VQBN, Nga TP, Le VL. Biosynthesis of silver nanoparticles using nanocurcumin extracted from fresh turmeric of Vietnam. International Journal of Materials Research. 2022;**113**(9):776-784. DOI: 10.1515/ijmr-2021-8377

[29] Hoang VN, Le XH, Pham NT, Vu DC, Le VV, Phan TD, et al. Fabrication and vibration characterization of curcumin extracted from turmeric (Curcuma longa) rhizomes of the northern Vietnam. Springerplus. 2016;**5**(1):1147. DOI: 10.1186/s40064-016-2812-2

[30] Nguyen DT, Nguyen TT, Nguyen TLN, Ho TP. The ability of ginger rhizome (Zingiber officinale Rosc) extract in producing of silver nanoparticles and the antibacterial activity of these nanoparticles. VNU Journal of Science: Natural Sciences and Technology. 2019;**35**(3):118-127. DOI: 10.25073/2588-1140/vnunst.4922

Chapter 4

Unexpected Results with New Homeopathic Complexes: A Review

Dorly de Freitas Buchi, Edvaldo S. Trindade and Carolina C. de Oliveira

Abstract

Despite homeopathy being a therapy that has been around for over 200 years, it still arouses controversy, both because of the high dilutions in which it is administered and because of the methodologies used in research, which are not always adequate to reach a definitive conclusion. Our group has been researching the action of single homeopathic products and homeopathic complexes on immune system cells and on tumor cells, both animal and human, for over 25 years. In this chapter, we intend to summarize the main results obtained in theses and dissertations, products of academic research with strict controls, all carried out by nonhomeopathic professionals, mainly by biologists and biochemists, whose conclusion is unquestionable. We may not know the detailed mechanisms of action of homeopathy, just as we do not know about most allopathic medicines, medicines that often work one way in a patient. In some people, the doses must be tested, or even sometimes have a paradoxical action in others. The results were surprising, and here we will present two of the investigated complexes, which have already been published with different names or acronyms, but which, in recent years, have been referred to as M1 (mixture 1) and M8 (mixture 8), letters and numbers used in a large double-blind study conducted.

Keywords: immune system, homeopathic complexes, macrophages, tumor cells, cytokines

1. Introduction

The growing popularity of complementary and alternative medicine in the public sector is reflected in the scientific community by an increase in the number of scientific papers attempting to assess the efficacy of therapeutic effects. Data on biological effects of ultra-dilutions are investigated with laboratory studies under carefully controlled conditions. The use of models with plants or animals allows the observation of direct responses, which eliminates subjectivity and speculation regarding to placebo effect, which is the main criticism in relation to studies with humans. The lack of conclusive studies that provide information on how homeopathy works, led us to test some homeopathic medicines, widely used by homeopathic physicians, using macrophages as biological models, as well as other cell types. To find out which medicine to look for, we held a meeting with homeopathic physicians with extensive clinical experience, asking which quick results suggested action on macrophages or other cells of the immune system. We were informed that some medications are even suggested as first aid, acting first on the symptoms, for example, pain and fever, and then they look for the "background medication." These drugs were exactly the ones we were interested in. These medicines were tested in macrophages culture, individually and mixed. These cells responded to all products, and surprisingly differently for each product. The results with *Mercurius solubilis* were the only one of the published single drugs [1]. The more interesting result is that *Merc sol* stimulated different macrophages answer, modulating the liberation of cytokines and reactive species production. Lower dilutions increase interferon-gamma (IFNγ), while the higher ones augmented IL-4 production after *in vitro* treatment. It should be noted that IFNγ promotes Th1 cell responses and IL-4 leads to Th2-type humoral immunity and is involved in proliferation and differentiation of activated B-cells. That is, the same substance but in different dilutions present paradoxical responses, which before being published, were repeated several times.

Returning to the complexes, that is also too interesting, not all mixtures worked; for example, when we added *Viscum album* or Turmeric (*Curcuma longa*), the complexes seem to be inactivated. The homeopathic extracts used to produce M1 and M8 were specified by name and by doses in **Table 1.**

It is known that cell cultures are particularly appropriate as an initial screening system in pharmaceutical research when possible modulatory effects of novel drugs are estimated. This experimental model seems to be particularly useful in evaluating

Composition	**Matrix**	**Final concentration (v/v%)**		
		M1	**M8**	
Aconitum napellus	MT	20 d	20 d	0.1×10^{-19}
Arsenicum album	6 d	18 d	18 d	0.1×10^{-17}
Asa foetida	MT	20 d	20 d	0.1×10^{-19}
Calcarea carbonica	8 d	16 d	16 d	0.1×10^{-15}
Chelidonium majus	MT	20 d	-	0.1×10^{-19}
Cinnamon	MT	20 d	-	0.1×10^{-19}
Conium maculatum	5 d	17 d	17 d	0.1×10^{-16}
Echinacea purpurea	MT	20 d	-	0.1×10^{-19}
Gelsemium sempervirens	MT	20 d	-	0.1×10^{-19}
Ipecacuanha	5 d	13 d	13 d	0.1×10^{-12}
Phosphorus	12 d	20 d	20 d	0.1×10^{-19}
Rhus toxicodendron	6 d	17 d	17 d	0.1×10^{-16}
Silicea	12 d	20 d	20 d	0.1×10^{-19}
Sulfur	12 d	24 d	24 d	0.1×10^{-23}
Thuja occidentalis	6 d	19 d	19 d	0.1×10^{-18}

Table 1.
Summary of the main differences between cytokines production and the treatment with M1 and M8 complexes. Tumor necrosis factor alpha (TNFα), when in excess, is more reduced by M8, interferon-gamma (IFNγ) is more reduced by M1, and interleukin 10 (IL-10) is enhanced by M1 and reduced by M8.

the effects of homeopathic treatments, due to the great possibility of data for statistical analysis, without the disadvantages of clinical screening.

The immune system works perfectly by coordinating actions between cells and proteins to provide defense against infection. These cells and proteins do not form a single organ like the heart or liver. Instead, the immune system is dispersed throughout the body to provide rapid responses to a possible invasion and infection. The development of all immune system cells begins in the bone marrow with a hematopoietic (blood-forming) stem cell. Although all components of the immune system interact with each other, it is typical to consider two broad categories of immune responses: the innate immune system and the adaptive immune system.

Innate immune responses are carried out without prior additional "training" to do their jobs. These cells include neutrophils, monocytes, natural killer (NK) cells, and a set of proteins termed complement proteins. Innate responses to infection occur rapidly and reliably. Adaptive immune responses comprise the second category. These responses involve T-cells and B-cells, two cell types that require "training" or education to learn not to attack our own cells. The advantages of adaptive responses are their long-lived memory and the ability to adapt to new germs. Activation of macrophages represents one of the first events in the innate response. The mechanisms of innate and adaptive immunity are, however, interdependent. This intercommunication is also performed through macrophages, which participate in the production, mobilization, activation, and regulation of all effector cells of the immune system. They interact reciprocally with other cells, which causes the change of their properties, for specialized immunological functions. Macrophages have an important role in the secretion of various cytokines, in addition to act as antigen-presenting cells (APCs).

Cytokines are produced by many cell populations, but the main producers are helper T (Th) cells and macrophages, which predominantly produce proinflammatory cytokines when activated, involved in the upregulation of inflammatory reactions. The anti-inflammatory cytokines are a series of immunoregulatory molecules that control the proinflammatory cytokine response. These specific cytokines or antagonists would act to disrupt the hyperexcitability cycle, providing a new, nonopioid therapeutic approach for the treatment of pathological pain due to inflammation or injury. Several situations can lead to systemic inflammatory syndromes in the human body. Their common feature is a massive release of cytokines due to excessive activation of immune cells. Cytokine storm is usually understood to mean an exacerbated immune response characterized by the release of cytokines and other mediators. These mediators are part of an evolutionarily well-conserved innate immune response that is required for the efficient elimination of infectious agents and the repair processes immediately. In an appropriate inflammatory response, there is a balance between adequate cytokine production to clear invaders, on the one hand, and avoidance of a hyperinflammatory response follows. A balanced, "protective" inflammatory response consists of diverse mechanisms and involves activation of both pro- and anti-inflammatory pathways within the innate and the acquired immune systems. You can see a good review of storm cytokines in Jarczak and Nierhaus [2].

Our laboratory at the Federal University of Paraná used to research the action of pesticides (agriculture is one of the strong points in our state and in the country), fungal and lichen extracts on tumor cells, macrophages, and the immune system in general. At the end of the 1990s, the positive pulmonary response found in some patients with the use of homeopathic products aroused our curiosity. As we already had a cell culture laboratory, we consulted health homeopaths professionals, and we established protocols. Despite homeopathy being a medical and pharmaceutical specialty in our country, it is still a therapy that raises much debate, often confused with belief, as if it were a religion. It is common to hear expressions like "I believe" or "I don't believe" in homeopathy.

Once we started to obtain quick and interesting answers, previous results were presented at conferences, and the questions asked by our peers led us to improve methodology to reduce possible variables. And curiosity led us to test different mixed products (homeopathic complexes) on cells and animals, but always produced according to the homeopathic pharmacopeia, by a specialized pharmacist. Highly diluted natural complexes comprise a combination of different compounds considered useful for a particular symptom or disease. The studies were double-blind, and positive and negative control groups were rigorously evaluated. The results were surprising with different products, but two of these complexes, due to their fast action, were studied more and became known by us as M1 and M8, symbols encoded in a double-blind study.

2. Methodology

In general, the evaluations were carried out in the following order: (1) first, *in vitro*, where mice or humans cells were treated with different potencies of a drug and evaluated morphologically; (2) still *in vitro*, the tests were repeated for metabolic and biochemical evaluations in the potencies that presented the most interesting results; (3) then, tumor cells from mice and humans were evaluated in the presence of treated immune cells; (4) finally, the mice were treated *in vivo* with the drugs in the potencies that showed the best results; at the end of the treatment, their cells were collected to be evaluated morphologically and biochemically; (5) finally, tumor cells were inoculated into the mice, which were then treated, the tumors collected and evaluated.

The results presented here were obtained from theses, dissertations, and published articles. Therefore, equipment and technologies used in conventional research and fundamental software were used, such as Mirax Viewer Software, ImageJ (NIH) Software, and ImageJ's Image Deconvolution plugin. The evaluations were done by light microscopy, confocal microscopy, transmission and scanning electron microscopy, flow cytometry, immunocytochemical, ultrastructural cytochemistry, invasion assay with transwell plates, human colon-rectal cancer cells stably transfected with the pNF-κB-hrGFP PlasmidStratagene was performed on HT-29 cells, histopathology, immunohistochemistry, ultrastructural pathology, slide scanning system, Microarrays and Gene Chips, microplate reader, enzyme-linked immunosorbent assay (ELISA), and many other routine biochemical techniques.

3. Main results and discussion

All homeopathic products we test must be shaken vigorously (succussion) before use. Whatever happens to the solution during shaking remains for a limited time.

Cell culture is a good technique to evaluate metabolic and morphologic changing by treatment with different drugs. In our lab, it was well-established immune and tumor cell culture. Macrophages are cells from the immune system whose response usually appears quickly since they are part of our body's first line of defense. The majority, around 80% of cells in the culture, changed morphology after internal and external treatment to an activated cell appearance, as observed by light or electron microscopy. In **Figure 1,** it is possible to observe morphologic modifications that macrophages presented after just 24 hours of treatment with our homeopathic products using different methodologies.

Studies in our lab demonstrated that homeopathic products activated macrophages both *in vivo* and *in vitro*. In addition, tumor necrosis factor-α (TNF α), when occurred excessive production *in vitro,* was significantly decreased [3]. It was observed by ultrastructural cytochemistry that NAD(P)H oxidase activity was increased as well as that of inducible nitric oxide synthase (iNOS), consequently producing reactive oxygen species (ROS) and nitric oxide (NO), respectively. NO inhibited cytochrome oxidase and peroxisomes activities. In response to stimuli, these cells underwent an activation that allowed them, among other functions, to acquire a great capacity to defeat microorganisms and some tumor cells. This can occur through oxygen or nitrogen-dependent mechanisms, in which reactive oxygen (ROS) and nitrogen (RNS) species are produced [4]. These diffuse and short-lived products have a role in

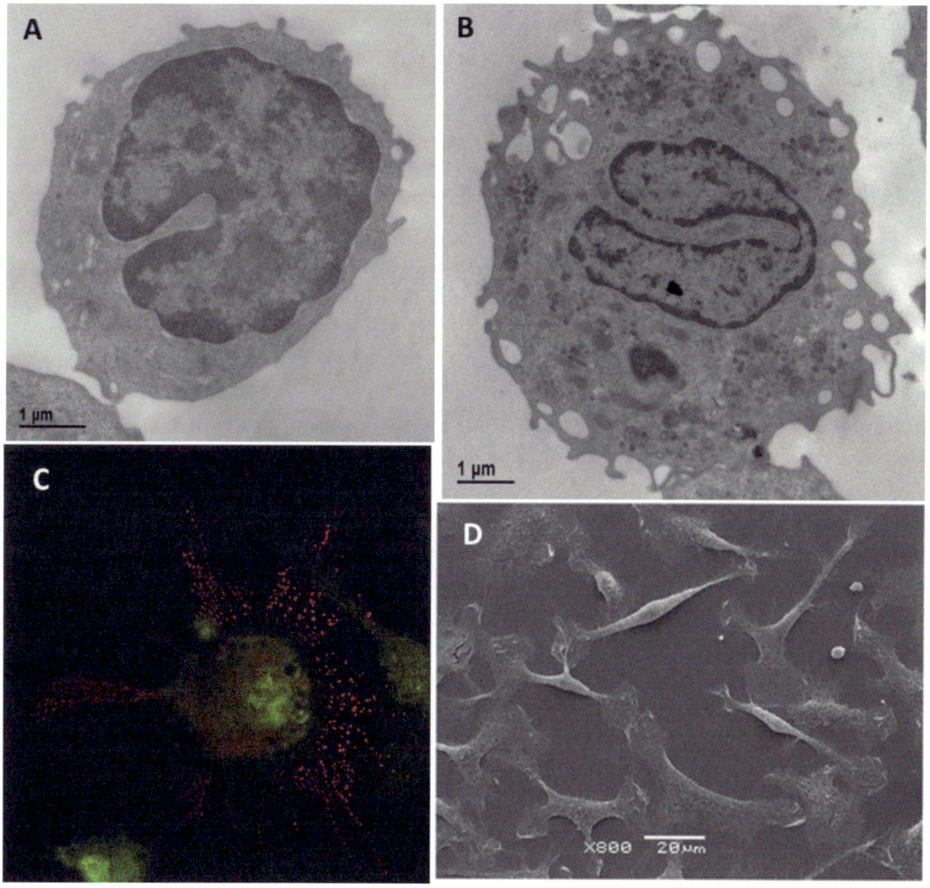

Figure 1.
Macrophages were observed by transmission (A and B), confocal (C), and scanning (D) electron microscopy. In A: resting macrophage, nucleus with condensed chromatin, and few cytoplasmic vesicles indicating only basal metabolism. B: activated macrophage with many euchromatins, cytoplasmatic vesicles, and projections suggesting high metabolism. In C: treated macrophage treated stained with Acridine Orange, showing acid vesicles in red and DNA in green at confocal microscopy. In D: a culture of treated macrophages with activated aspect, most of them sprayed.

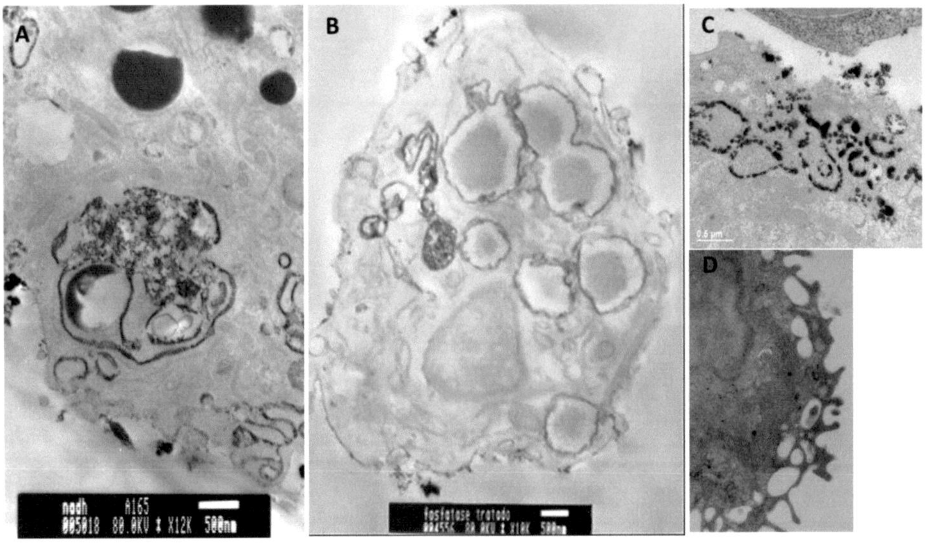

Figure 2.
Ultrastructural images of macrophage enzymes. Treated macrophages showed an increase of endosomal/lysosomal system in transmission electron microscopy. The ultrastructural cytochemistry showed cells labeled with cerium chloride for different enzymes. In A, the vesicles showed NAD(P)H oxidase activity; in B, they were labeled for acid phosphatase; in C, the vesicles were labeled for Mg++ATPase; in D, cytochrome oxidase activity (the one that decreased the activity). These cells were observed without contrasting with lead, avoiding possible contaminants.

antimicrobial defense, which are well-defined and signaled in the cell. For the protection of macrophages against these toxic products, ROS are stored in vesicles called lysosomes, which can be placed in contact with vesicles that contain the ingested material, the phagosomes, or endosomes. In **Figure 2,** it is possible to observe the cellular vesicles labeled by cerium chloride for different membrane cytoplasmatic enzymes. To make sure that the label is the result of cerium chloride precipitation after the activity of the respective enzyme, these cells were not stained with lead or uranyl. After treatment, the cells showed an increase of endosomal/lysosomal system, amplifying the capacity to phagocyte noninfective microorganisms and cell debris [5]. All these metabolic alterations were those we could measure. But we can ask, how many other alterations occur? How many alterations do we not have technology to measure yet and are occurring not only in macrophages but also in other cells? We tested in macrophages because we know that these cells are extremely sensitive to small modifications in their microenvironment, thus being able to successfully perform its various functions. In the scheme represented in **Figure 3**, we can summarize its main functions in the control of other cells of the immune system, modifying the inflammatory response, healing, cellular, humoral defense, etc.

Physical and chemical barriers, such as skin and mucosal surfaces, limit microorganisms to the body's outer surfaces, and when pathogens can break down, these barriers are usually destroyed by the immune system. Thanks to this system, animals can resist almost all types of microorganisms or toxins that tend to damage tissues and organs and even often protect us from infections and modified cells such as cancer cells. As part of the natural body response, inflammation is a complex process that includes a variety of cells and molecules such as the immune cells and cytokines as mediators. Its function is mainly focused on eliminating the injury cause, clearing out damaged cells and tissues, and initiating tissue repair. Therefore, inflammation

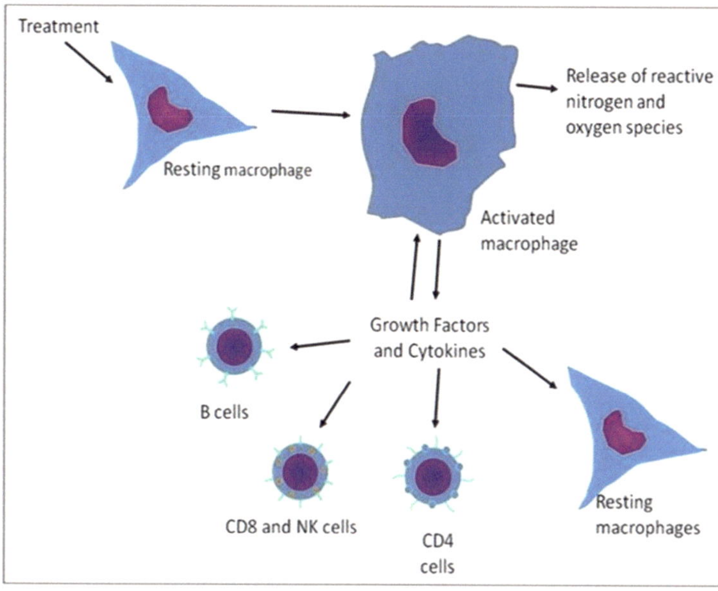

Figure 3.
After 60 days of infection, the lesions of the control BALB/c mice, treated orally with the vehicle, developed progressive centrally located crusts, exhibiting an ulcerative pattern. In the M1-treated group, the lesions caused by the parasites developed slower than the control, presenting reduced paw thickness. There was edema in the early lesions, followed by almost complete remission of the lesion.

is considered as a mechanism of innate immunity. Old names for cytokines are lymphokines, interleukins, and chemokines. An inflammatory cytokine or proinflammatory cytokine is a type of signaling molecule that is excreted from immune cells (not only) that promote inflammation and play an important role in mediating the innate immune response. Inflammatory cytokines are predominantly produced by and involved in the upregulation of inflammatory reactions. The anti-inflammatory cytokines are a series of immunoregulatory molecules that control the proinflammatory cytokine response. The main function of cytokine receptors is to convert an extracellular signal, such as a specific binding of a cytokine to a target cell, into an intracellular signal, such as the activation of an enzyme or a transcription factor that can trigger a response of the target cell. Treatment alone did not change cytokines production by cells, but when cells were stimulated with lipopolysaccharide (LPS) and then treated, IFN-γ and TNF-α production was decreased.

Tumor necrosis factor alpha (TNF-α) is an important inflammatory factor that acts as a master switch in establishing an intricate link between inflammation and cancer. TNF-α secretion can be induced by conserved structural elements common to microbial pathogens as well as by tumor cells. Several studies have focused on the transcriptional regulation of TNF-α, looking at transcription factors that bind to the responsive element sites within the TNF-α promoter. NF-κB is a transcription factor that plays crucial roles in inflammation and immunity. Many proinflammatory stimuli can activate NF-κB, mainly through IKK-dependent phosphorylation and degradation of the IκB inhibitory proteins. When NF-κB translocates to the nucleus, it activates the transcription of target genes, including cytokines like TNF-α, chemokines, and antiapoptotic factors [6]. We have used a reporter cell line, HT29-pNF-κB-hrGFP, to find out if M1, M2, and M8, in the presence or absence of TNF-α stimulus,

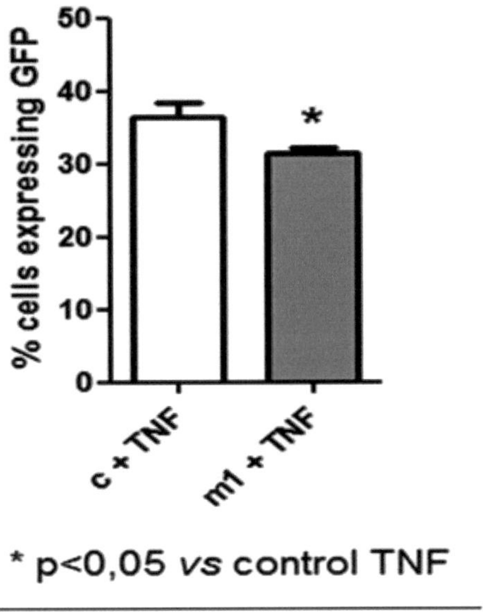

Figure 4.
HT-29 cell line (human carcinoma colon-rectal cells) transfected with plasmid pNF-κB-hrGFP showed a reduction in NF-kb complex activation after 48 h of treatment with M1 (In collaboration with institute Pasteur—Montevideo—Uruguay).

have any effect on NF-κB activity. The reporter cell line HT29-pNF-κB-hrGFP is routinely used to screen natural or synthetic compounds that interfere and/or modulate NF-κB activity. HT29 cells were stimulated for 24 h with a proinflammatory cocktail. GFP (green fluorescent protein) positive cells were sorted. We have observed that only M1 has decreased NF-κB activity on TNF-α stimulated HT29-pNF-κB-hrGFP cells. Thus, we tested *in vitro* different M1 concentrations (10, 20, ad 30%) and they all presented the same effect on NF-κB activity [3]. We have observed that only M1 has decreased NF-κB activity (**Figure 4**), but it was not downregulated by M2 and M8. However, we have observed TNF-α reduction by these highly diluted tinctures.

Leishmaniasis is a disease that produces high morbidity but low mortality and results in stigma-producing deformities. In the Americas, it is caused mainly by *Leishmania* sp, and requires treatment. The parasite is of great medical and veterinary public health significance, for it infects numerous mammal species, including humans. The parasites enter mammalian hosts through the bite of sandflies and replicate intracellularly. Cutaneous Leishmaniasis, the most common form of the disease, causes ulcers on exposed parts of the body, leading to disfigurement, permanent scars, stigma, and in some cases, disability. Modulatory effects were well observed in experimental infection, both *in vivo* and *in vitro,* by *L. amazonensis*, controlling infection progression and limiting its dissemination [7]. The animals were infected with parasites, and after 60 days, when the lesion was well-established, the animals were treated orally for 30 days. The treatment did not allow parasitic evolution as in the control animals. In **Figure 5**, it is possible to observe the difference in leishmaniosis lesions between animals treated or not. Probably among the slight metabolic changes that occur in the macrophages of treated mice is the increase in the production of Interleukin-10 (IL-10), considered an anti-inflammatory cytokine, the increase of ROS and NOS, and the increase in the number of natural killer cells (NK cells) by

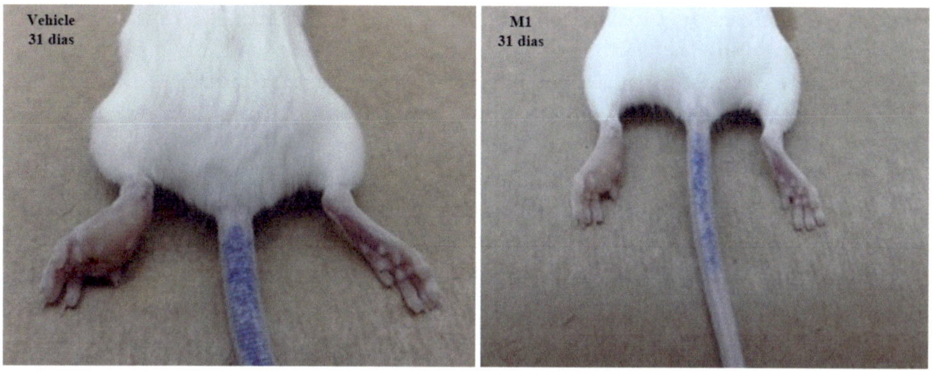

Figure 5.
Leishmaniosis amazonensis lesion: after 60 days of infection, the lesions of the control BALB/c mice, treated orally with the vehicle, developed progressive centrally located crusts, exhibiting an ulcerative pattern. In the M1-treated group, the lesions caused by the parasites were developed slower than the control, presenting reduced paw thickness. There was edema in the early lesions, followed by almost complete remission of the lesion.

treatment *in vitro* and *in vivo* with M1 are responsible for this impressive result. After the well-established lesion, the mice were treated with M1 for 30 days and we compare the evolution during the treatment. The evolution of lesions during this 30 days on the footpad of mice paws infected with the parasite *Leishmania amazonensis* can be seen in **Figure 6**. Note that M1 decreases the progression of the lesion throughout the treatment and shows a statistical difference after 30 days (* $p < 0.05$). Each point represents the average of five animals per group.

Beyond increasing ROS and NOS, the M1 complex also increased the number of natural killer (NK) cells and their activity. Cells of the innate immune system recognize pathogens and tissue injury. The processes are rapid, nonspecific, and include

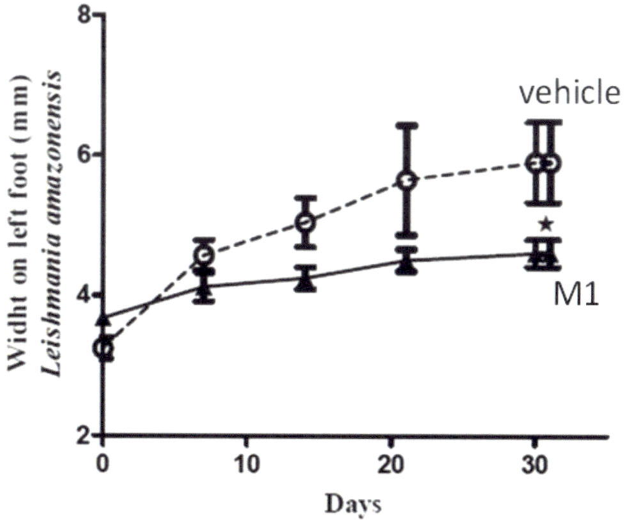

Figure 6.
Evolution of lesions on the footpad of mice paws infected with the parasite Leishmania amazonensis: the mice were treated with M1 for 30 days and compared here with the control group that was treated with water (H_2O). Note that M1 decreases the progression of the lesion throughout the treatment and shows a statistical difference after 30 days ($p < 0.05$). Each point represents the average of five animals per group.*

responses such as phagocytosis, cell locomotion, killing of pathogens or cells, and cytokine production. These innate immune mechanisms are usually very effective in the elimination of invading pathogens because NK cells can recognize the target cell without the need to be activated by prior immunization or stimulation by contact with antigen-presenting cells as occurs in T-cells to become efficient in their response. Since their identification in 1975, NK cells have been classified as lymphocytes based on their morphology, expression of lymphocyte markers, and their common origin from lymphoid progenitor cells in the bone marrow. NK cells, however, are generally considered components of the innate immune defense because they do not need antigen-specific receptors on their surface to carry out their activities. Their derivation from either lymphoid or myeloid lineages was debated early in their discovery. Research showed that NK cells can be derived from common lymphoid progenitors, and some studies have shown that progenitors expressing myeloid antigens can also develop into NK cells. However, alternative views have been proposed, including the existence of a common myeloid-lymphoid progenitor and this process depending on which cytokines they are exposed. The notion that myeloid precursors previously known to give rise to monocyte/macrophage and Dendritic Cells (DCs) are also capable of NK-cell differentiation puts the recent findings in a new therapeutic perspective. Therefore, NK cells are innate immune effector cells [8, 9].

Our group also performed assays to evaluate *in vitro* effects of M1 in a coculture model between human mononuclear cells obtained from leukoreduction chambers (LRS chambers) after plateletpheresis procedure and melanoma cells. When mononuclear cells were analyzed by flow cytometry, an increase in CD3−/CD56+ natural killer cell population was observed in the treated group. Finally, after treatment, when isolated from mononuclear cultures, and co-cultured with human metastatic melanoma cell lineage, those natural killer cells from M1 treated group revealed a significantly increased cytotoxicity against melanoma cells (**Figure** 7) [3]. This occurred only with M1 treatment.

The immune system, a set of defense and healing mechanisms of our body, is highly competent and controlled, performing its functions without compromising

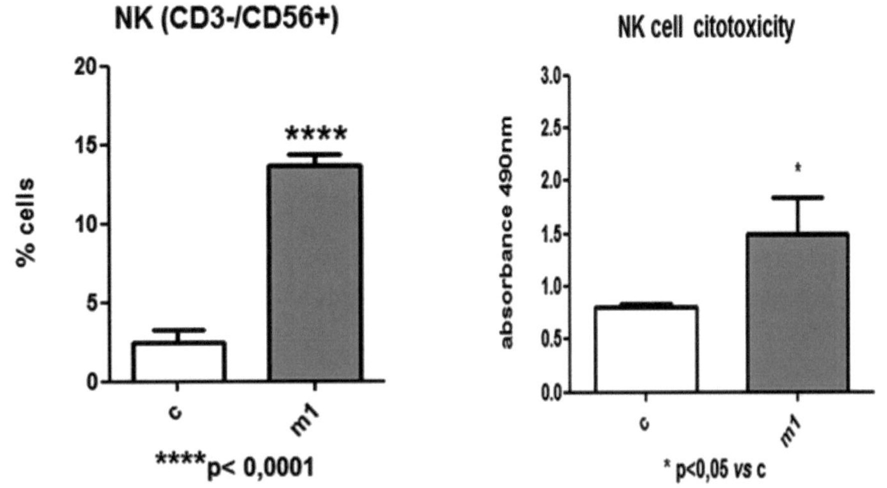

Figure 7.
Detection of CD3 and CD56 markers (natural killer cells) by flow cytometry in a population of mononuclear cells after coculture with 1205Lu tumor cells. After co-cultivation, mononuclear cells previously treated (48 h) with the M1 complex showed a statistically significant increase in the percentage of CD3−/CD56+ (NK) cells.

the rest of the body. However, many autoimmune diseases, immunodepression syndromes, and cancer may be the result of disorders in the immune system, where the action of this decisively determines the patient's prognosis, and an inadequate or insufficient immune response can mean the loss of the body's fight against the disease. In these cases, why not rehabilitate it and stimulate it to perform its function, guiding it to eliminate the disease? Unlike the drugs used by allopathic medicine, which act directly on the physiological processes related to disease symptoms, homeopathic medicines promote the individual improvement of a general health state, stimulating the immune system to trigger appropriate responses for each situation. Thus, homeopathic treatment allows the individual to restore health and prevent disease without, however, producing the side effects experienced by many of the conventional treatments. The incredible adaptability and intelligence of the immune system, which keeps us healthy, despite considerable adversities, is crucial. It is important to note that the existence of this force that works to keep us as healthy as possible was perceived and accepted before we know the cells and molecules that make up the immune system.

Cytokines are soluble, low molecular-weight proteins that mediate cell-to-cell communication. They can modulate the host immune response toward cancer cells and induce apoptosis. Cytokine-based immunotherapy has been a promising area of research and is currently an area of much interest, mainly due to the large amount of side effects. That is why there is a lot of discussion about the burden and bonus balance of its use. You can see a good revision in [10]. Cancer cells, despite their phenotypic characteristics acquired by genetic and epigenetic alterations, do not act alone in the development of the disease. Cancer-associated fibroblasts are involved in all the processes leading to physiological changes that allow cancer cells to become malignant, such as the production of extracellular matrix molecules and its remodeling, providing survival signals, and promoting cancer cell invasion and proliferation. Gonçalves and Potrich [11] used molecular biology techniques and standard functional assays to assess the changes related to the metastatic phenotype. The findings of this study indicate that these products reprogram, molecularly and functionally, melanoma cells *in vitro*, modulating their metastatic phenotype [11]. Guimaraes et al. [12] described the results of an experimental laboratory validation of the potential of peritoneal macrophages, challenged with a complex homeopathic medication (CHM/M8), to stimulate the immune effectiveness of mesenteric lymph node lymphocytes. This new form of immunomodulatory therapy is based on Hahnemann's ancient homeopathic techniques, which use diluted substances that are vigorously shaken (succussed) during preparation. The results of this kind of treated coculture were fast and treated macrophages and lymphocytes exhibited a greater degree of interaction than did control cells. Evidence of tumor cells in apoptosis induced by stimulated lymphocytes, apparently prevented tumor cells could use their multiple mechanisms to escape of the immune system. Such findings are likely to be responsible for the attenuation of tumor growth and lung colonization previously observed *in vivo* [12–14].

If we collected the supernatant of treated macrophage culture and added it to lymphocytes culture, these lymphocytes could destroy melanoma cells [12]. It is important to note that those lymphocytes could not do this before the treatment. When melanoma cells were injected into mice veins to cause lung melanoma nodules, and the animals inhaled M8 for only 2 weeks, the number of nodules was reduced [13]. When the tumor cells were inoculated in the dorsal subcutaneous region, a solid tumor mass was developed, but after 2 weeks of inhalation, the tumor mass was smaller than the control one, showing that inhalation for only two weeks did not

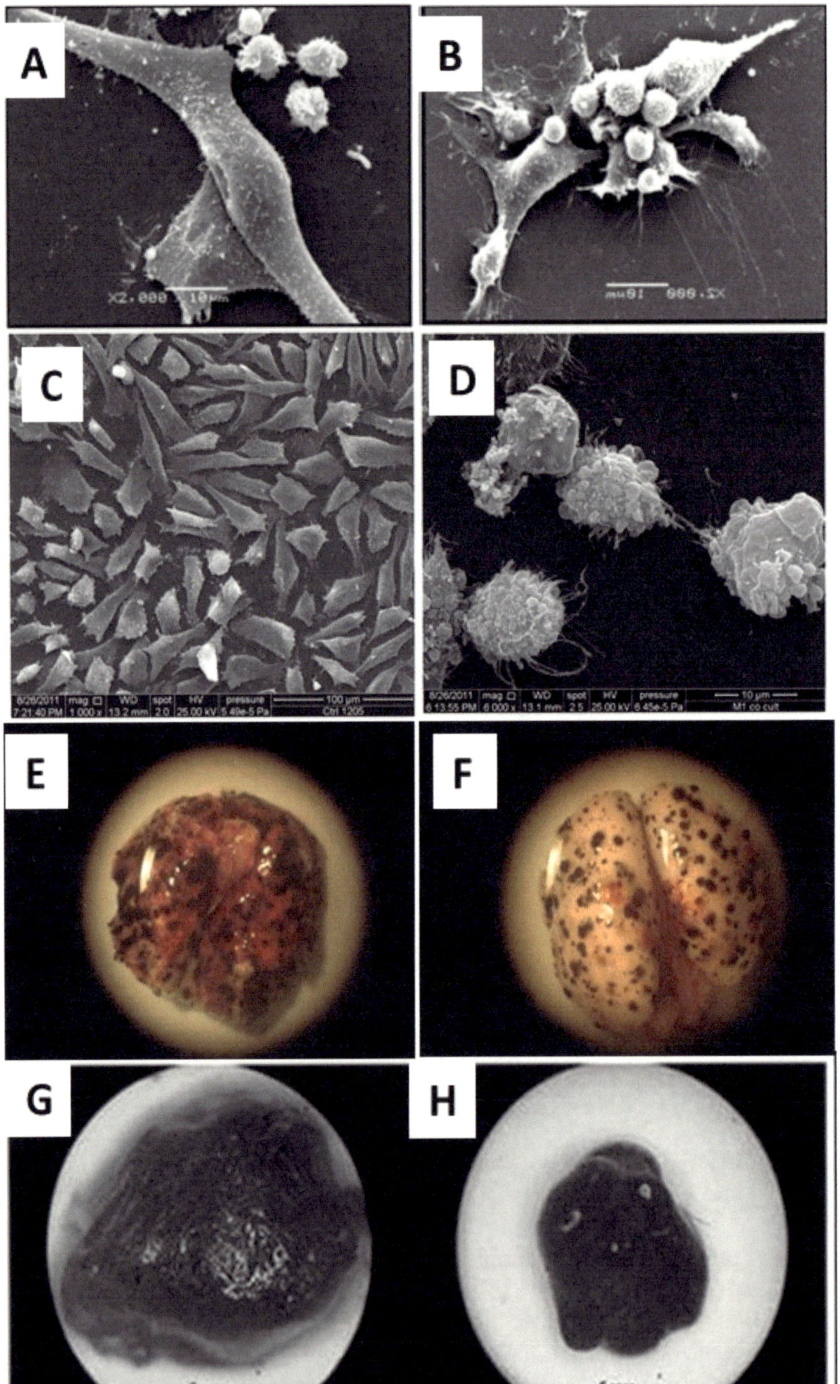

Figure 8.
Images of mice and human melanoma cells, and mice tumor nodules and tumor mass after treatment with the homeopathic complexes. At left-A, C, E, and G control groups; images at right-treated groups. A and B: the big cell melanoma cells in culture; the small one, lymphocytes. C and D: human melanoma cells in culture, and in D dying cells after adding treated lymphocytes; E and F lungs with melanoma nodules; G and H tumor mass. A–D, cells observed at scanning electron microscopy; E–H at light microscopy.

allow tumor mass to grow in the same velocity (**Figure 8**) [14]. If you think that the animals did not have defense against the millions of tumor cells inoculated, it was an amazing and fast defense answer. More about answers of immune system cells and inflammation after treatment with homeopathy in [15].

4. Conclusion

The activation of macrophages represents one of the first events in the innate response. The mechanisms of innate and adaptive immunity are, however, interdependent. This intercommunication is also carried out through macrophages, which participate in the production, mobilization, activation, and regulation of all effector cells in the immune system. They interact reciprocally with other cells, which causes their properties to change, for specialized immune functions. Macrophages play an important role in the secretion of various cytokines in addition to acting as antigen-presenting cells. The results of our research have shown that homeopathic medicines stimulate the immune system to trigger appropriate responses for each situation and do not produce side effects. The development of therapies capable of modulating the inflammatory process, without suppressing the desirable effect of its physiological aspects, could be an interesting alternative to obtain a better efficacy of the tissue response against external aggressors. We are sure that much more studies will be needed to verify the effects of homeopathy on diseased organisms. But we are also sure that highly diluted drugs that act on isolated cells in a cell culture are not having a placebo effect, since careful controls were performed during all experiments.

The harmonic results obtained in research during these years allowed us to conclude that, in general, highly diluted products trigger quick and effective responses by living organisms, whether cells or animals, or people. M1 and M8 are homeopathic complex medicines with immunomodulatory properties, without toxicity or mutagenic effects. This homeopathic immunotherapy can restore the immune system to recognize tumors or infected cells; thus, it can be used to help some diseases without acting on a specific molecular target and without toxicity, since self-healing is stimulated through immune system. Here in **Table 2** we show the composition of M1 and M8 complexes. Therefore, the M1 and M8 complexes can be good candidates for complementary therapy to conventional treatments. Complementary does not mean one or the other, but that if you complement the conventional treatment with these products, you surely increase the chances of rehabilitation.

Homeopathy is a medical and pharmaceutical specialty and must be submitted to standard evaluation. Therefore, taking together all the results published, by using

Cytokines	M1	M8
TNF-α	↓	↓ ↓
IFN-γ	↑	↓ ↓
IL-10	↓	↓

Table 2.
Final composition of M1 and M8 (MT = Mother Tincture).

standard assays and methodologically reproducible tests verified by statistical analyses, we could demonstrate by scientific evidence that those homeopathic complexes presented effects on cellular and molecular levels. It is important to note that homeopathy is just another kind of treatment. These results show the importance of basic research in obtaining new knowledge about homeopathic medicine, using techniques and methods accepted by conventional medicine.

Acknowledgements

We are deeply grateful to all the people who have passed through our laboratories at Universidade Federal do Paraná, Brazil, whether for a simple internship, a postgraduation, or a postdoc. They had carried out the research carefully, with love, and often with the opposition from the academic community. They really are special people. We are also grateful to the research funding agencies CNPq, CAPES, and Paraná Tecnologia, to the Federal University of Paraná (UFPR) for unconditional support, and to the Electronic Microscopy Center of UFPR.

Competing interests

The authors declare that they have no competing interests.

Author details

Dorly de Freitas Buchi[1,2]*, Edvaldo S. Trindade[1] and Carolina C. de Oliveira[1]

1 Federal University of Paraná, Brazil

2 Bonaireswiss, Zürich, Switzerland

*Address all correspondence to: dorlybuchi@gmail.com

References

[1] Oliveira SM et al. Mercurius solubilis: Actions on macrophages. Homeopathy. 2011;**100**:228-236. DOI: 10.1016/j.homp.2011.05.005

[2] Jarczak D, Nierhaus A. Cytokine storm-Definition, causes, and implications. International Journal of Molecular Sciences. 2022;**23**:11740. DOI: 10.3390/ijms231911740

[3] De Oliveira CC et al. Developments on drug discovery and on new therapeutics: Highly diluted tinctures act as biological response modifiers. BMC Complementary and Alternative Medicine. 2011;**11**:101. Available from: http://www.biomedcentral.com/1472-6882/11/101

[4] De Oliveira CC et al. Canova, a Brazilian medical formulation, alters oxidative metabolism of mice macrophages. Journal of Infection. 2006;**52**(6):420-432

[5] Lopes L et al. Phagocytosis, endosomal/lysosomal system and other cellular aspects of macrophage activation by Canova medication. Micron. 2006;**37**(3):277-287. DOI: 10.1016/j.micron.2005.08.005

[6] Gilmore TD. The Rel/NF-kappaB signal transduction pathway: Introduction. Oncogene. 1999;**18**(49):684. DOI: 10.1038/sj.onc.1203237

[7] Nascimento KF et al. M1 homeopathic complex trigger effective responses against *Leishmania (L) amazonensis*. Cytokine. 2017;**99**:80-90. DOI: 10.1016/j.cyto.2017.07.001

[8] Laskowski TJ et al. Natural killer cells in antitumour adoptive cell immunotherapy. Nature, Reviews, Cancer. 2022;**22**:558. DOI: 10.1038/s41568-022-00491-0

[9] Wu SY et al. Natural killer cells in cancer biology and therapy. Molecular Cancer Review. 2020;**19**:120. DOI: 10.1186/s12943-020-01238-x

[10] Rallis SK et al. Cytokine-based cancer immunotherapy: Challenges and opportunities for IL-10. Anticancer Research. 2021;**41**:3247-3252. DOI: 10.21873/anticanres.15110

[11] Goncalves JP, Potrich FB, et al. In vitro attenuation of classic metastatic melanoma-related features by highly diluted natural complexes: Molecular and functional analyses. International Journal of Oncology. 2019;**55**:721-732. DOI: 10.3892/ijo.2019.4846

[12] Guimaraes FS et al. Stimulation of lymphocyte anti-melanoma activity by co-cultured macrophages activated by complex homeopathic medication. BMC Cancer. 2009;**9**:293. DOI: 10.1186/1471-2407-9-293

[13] Guimaraes FS et al. In vitro and in vivo anticancer properties of a Calcarea carbonica derivative complex (M8) treatment in a murine melanoma model. BMC Cancer. 2010;**10**:113. Available from: http://www.biomedcentral.com/1471-2407/10/113

[14] Andrade LF et al. Inhalation therapy with M1 inhibits experimental melanoma development and metastases in mice. Homeopathy. 2016;**105**(1):109-118. DOI: 10.1016/j.homp.2015.08.007

[15] Bellavite P et al. Immunology and homeopathy. 2. Cells of the immune system and inflammation. Evidence-based Complementary and Alternative Medicine. 2006;**3**(1):13-24. DOI: 10.1093/ecam/nek018

Chapter 5

Acupuncture Management in the Field of Assisted Reproductive Technology

Jie Yang, Liying Liu, Xiaoyan Zheng, Jingwen Zhang and Yuanyuan Lai

Abstract

Acupuncture is an ancient traditional Chinese medical practice that involves the insertion of fine needles into specific acupuncture points to rebalance energy and improve blood circulation within the body. Assisted reproductive technology (ART) is a method used to help couples who are unable to conceive naturally fulfill their desire for parenthood. Within ART, acupuncture management is utilized as adjunctive therapy to optimize the reproductive environment and increase the chances of a successful pregnancy. Acupuncture, as an adjunctive treatment modality in ART, offers unique advantages in regulating endocrine function, enhancing blood circulation, and reducing stress. Drawing upon a decade of experience in acupuncture-assisted reproduction and previous research, this chapter provides an overview of the clinical applications of acupuncture in different stages of ART and explores its potential mechanisms of action in the treatment of male infertility and female infertility. It highlights the promising prospects of acupuncture-like adjunctive therapies in the field of ART.

Keywords: acupuncture, assisted reproductive technology, *in vitro* fertilization, adjunctive treatment, complementary medicine

1. Introduction

Infertility refers to couples who have cohabited for at least a year and have a normal sexual life without using contraceptives but are still unable to conceive [1]. Statistically, between 8 and 12 percent of reproductive couples worldwide are infertile [2]. Since the first successful use of conventional in vitro fertilization (IVF) in 1978, assisted reproductive technology (ART) has rapidly evolved and become an important means of resolving infertility, which plays a crucial role in achieving fertility [3, 4]. ART, which includes artificial insemination (AI) and in vitro fertilization-embryo transfer (IVF-ET) and its derivatives, is a modern method for creating new life. IVF-ET involves egg donation, sperm donation, gestational carriers, ovarian stimulation, egg retrieval, embryo culture, and transfer [5, 6]. ART, the last resort if medications and surgery fail, had birthed over 8 million babies by 2020. Since reproductive medicine developed, the clinical pregnancy rate (CPR) has been 29–35% [7], whereas the live birth rate (LBR) is barely 30% [8].

As a treasure of Chinese medicine, acupuncture was accumulated through long-term medical practice by ancient people. It has the characteristics of safety, effectiveness, wide applicability, simplicity, and economy. Acupuncture has made great contributions to the prosperity and development of the Chinese nation for thousands of years and gradually plays a unique role in the world's healthcare industry. The treatment principle of acupuncture is mainly to stimulate the acupoints of the human body through various acupuncture instruments and special treatment techniques to adjust the balance of yin and yang, promote the circulation of qi and blood, and accelerate the circulation of the meridians. Compared with other treatment methods, acupuncture has obvious advantages in the comprehensive treatment of local and systemic conditions. It can be said that the essence of acupuncture action is to initiate, promote, and adjust, rather than supplement and intervene with exogenous substances.

Acupuncture has a long history as a safe and effective physical therapy with few side effects in the treatment of infertility. In 1999, Stener-Victorin and their colleagues [9] were the first to find that electroacupuncture (EA) benefits embryo implantation, and women's pregnancy in the process of ART and can relieve the pain of patients during oocyte retrieval. Since then, studying how and why acupuncture makes ART work better has become an important area of research in this field. Several studies have investigated the mechanisms of acupuncture in male or female infertility. For instance, acupuncture affects the female reproductive endocrine immune system by activating the hypothalamic–pituitary-ovarian (HPO) axis [10]. EA can improve sperm function by increasing the functional expression of CatSper corporate channels in sperm [11].

With our wealth of expertise gained from ten years of experience in acupuncture-assisted reproduction and extensive prior research, this chapter offers a comprehensive examination of acupuncture's clinical applications throughout various stages of ART. It delves into the potential mechanisms underlying acupuncture's efficacy in addressing both male and female infertility while emphasizing the optimistic outlook for acupuncture-related complementary therapies in the realm of ART.

2. Clinical research for acupuncture management in the ART process

As the demand for safe and holistic approaches to improve fertility outcomes continues to grow, clinical research investigating the efficacy of acupuncture in the management of ART procedures has become paramount. By examining the available evidence, we aim to provide a comprehensive overview of the current understanding of acupuncture's potential benefits and its impact on key aspects of the ART journey, including controlled ovarian hyperstimulation (COH), oocyte quality, embryo transfer, pregnancy rates, etc. The overall outlooks of clinical research for acupuncture management in ART were shown in **Figure 1**.

2.1 Acupuncture management during the COH

COH is a medical procedure employed in ART to induce the development of multiple follicles in the ovaries, thereby increasing the likelihood of successful pregnancy for women undergoing IVF or other ART procedures. Significant advancements in

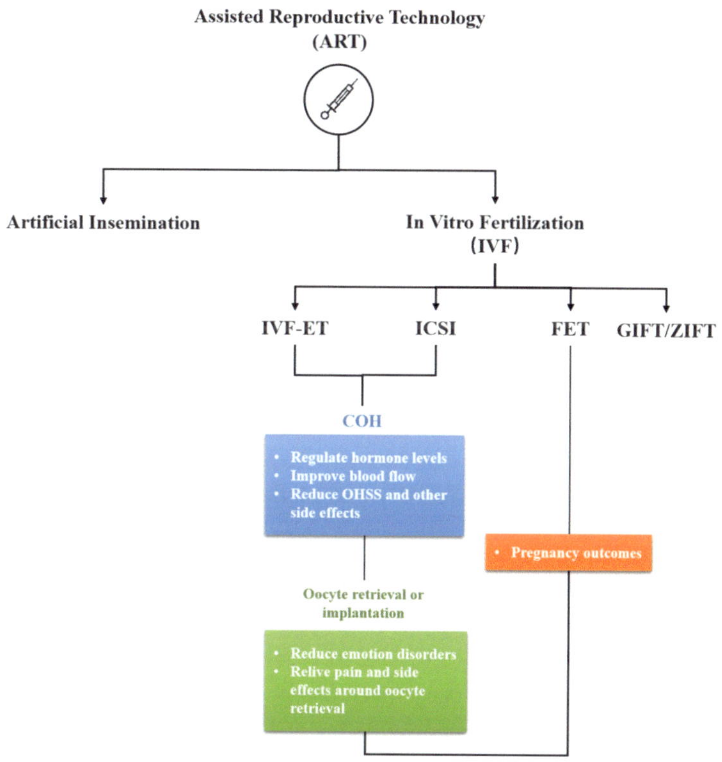

Figure 1.
The overall outlooks of clinical research for acupuncture management in ART.

COH programs have been achieved, primarily driven by the research and development of innovative therapeutic agents. However, it has become evident that overly aggressive ovarian management can have detrimental effects on a woman's reproductive system. COH can lead to the occurrence of side effects, such as ovarian hyperstimulation syndrome (OHSS). To address these concerns, acupuncture has emerged as a valuable approach for managing the symptoms associated with COH and OHSS. By stimulating the body's innate healing mechanisms and promoting relaxation, acupuncture offers a complementary therapy to alleviate the adverse effects.

2.1.1 Regulate hormone levels

Acupuncture has been shown to stimulate the production of endorphins, which can help regulate hormone levels and improve reproductive function. As early as 2009, a study found that the regulation of cortisol and prolactin in the acupuncture group appeared to be beneficial during the medication phase of IVF treatment, with a trend toward a more normal fertility cycle dynamic [12]. Poor ovarian response (POR) to ovarian stimulation usually indicates a reduction in follicular response, resulting in a reduced number of retrieved oocytes [13]. Based on our newly published systematic review, we found that acupuncture treatment during COH is questionable in improving pregnancy outcomes in POR patients. However, acupuncture can increase sex hormone levels and improve ovarian function in women with POR [14, 15].

2.1.2 Improve blood flow

Acupuncture can improve blood flow to the uterus and ovaries, which can improve the chances of success in ART procedures. Transvaginal Doppler ultrasonography advances the pathophysiological understanding of female pelvic hemodynamics [16]. The latest Doppler indices differed significantly between women with and without ovarian dysfunction and correlated significantly with markers of ovarian dysfunction, and these results support the use of Doppler ultrasound to detect ovarian dysfunction [17]. Patients undergoing IVF have a Doppler ultrasound of the uterine arteries before the day of egg retrieval, a test that is thought to be associated with success after embryo transfer [18]. Positive effects of acupuncture for infertility may be related to endorphin system inhibition of central sympathetic nerves, altered uterine blood flow and motility, and stress reduction [19].

Our previous study found a trend toward relatively high doses of acupuncture to have better results in women with poor endometrial receptivity and to significantly improve the uterine blood flow (UBF) index in this type of patient [20]. The latest study also confirms our view and recommends acupuncture as an intervention to improve UBF [21, 22]. In addition, our systematic review of studies related to the improvement of ovarian blood flow by acupuncture included 20 studies with 1611 participants of luteinized unruptured follicle syndrome, polycystic ovary syndrome (PCOS), poor ovarian insufficient (POI), premature ovarian failure (POF), and diminished ovarian reserve (DOR) patients, found acupuncture could significantly improve the ovary blood flow (OBF) parameters, including vascular resistance index and peak systolic velocity (PSV).

2.1.3 Reduce OHSS and other side effects

Acupuncture possesses noteworthy anti-inflammatory properties, rendering it beneficial in mitigating the occurrence of OHSS and countering other potential side effects associated with COH. By incorporating acupuncture into the treatment regimen, women with PCOS who undergo IVF or intracytoplasmic sperm injection (ICSI) can witness improvements in their CPR as well as ongoing pregnancy rate (OPR). Furthermore, acupuncture plays a crucial role in diminishing the risk of OHSS in this specific patient population, thereby contributing to a more favorable outcome in their assisted reproductive journey [23].

2.2 Acupuncture management around the time of oocyte retrieval or implantation

Acupuncture has demonstrated its effectiveness in alleviating mood disorders that may arise during the process of egg retrieval or transplantation, providing much-needed emotional support for patients. By incorporating acupuncture into pre- and post-procedural care, individuals undergoing these interventions can experience improvements in their overall mood and emotional well-being. Moreover, acupuncture also proves beneficial in mitigating the pain associated with the procedure, offering a non-invasive and natural approach to pain management. The strategic application of acupuncture techniques can help alleviate discomfort, reduce anxiety, and promote relaxation, thereby enhancing the overall experience for patients undergoing oocyte retrieval or transplantation.

2.2.1 Reduce emotion disorders

Multiple studies have substantiated the presence of elevated levels of state anxiety and depression in patients undergoing IVF, particularly during critical stages such as oocyte retrieval or embryo transfer [24]. It has been observed that this anxiety and depression tend to persist across multiple cycles of treatment. Encouragingly, a systematic evaluation conducted by Hullender Rubin, Smith et al. [25] indicates a noteworthy yet modest impact of acupuncture on reducing state anxiety specifically during oocyte retrieval or implantation, when compared to various control groups. Nevertheless, further high-quality evidence is essential to validate and strengthen these findings.

2.2.2 Relive pain and side effects around oocyte retrieval

We published a systematic review suggesting that acupuncture-combined analgesic therapy is more effective than utilizing conscious sedation and analgesia or non-steroidal anti-inflammatory drugs alone. In addition, there is no clear consensus on whether acupuncture applied alone during oocyte retrieval has analgesic effects, which requires further research [26]. Among these, EA is widely used for analgesia during oocyte retrieval with a mixed frequency and a fixed frequency for short-duration EA with similar analgesic effects [27, 28].

2.3 Acupuncture management for the pregnancy outcomes

Acupuncture has been used in various assisted reproductive technologies, including IVF-ET, frozen embryo transfer (FET), and ICSI, and studies have shown that acupuncture can improve biochemical and clinical pregnancies; however, no studies have yet shown that acupuncture can significantly improve LBR in patients undergoing assisted reproductive technologies. A randomized controlled study published in JAMA in 2018 showed that acupuncture was effective in improving LBRs before and after oocyte extraction or on and before and after ET, there were no overall benefits of acupuncture in improving LBRs when performed [29]. However, in two other systematic evaluations, acupuncture was found to improve clinical pregnancy during IVF [30, 31]. Another study confirmed that acupuncture before or during FET helped improve patients' biochemical pregnancy, and clinical pregnancy outcomes and the risk of serious adverse events is very low [32]. However, no significant improvement of acupuncture for live birth during FET was reported.

3. Mechanism of acupuncture treatment of female infertility

The etiology of female infertility is complex, including ovulation dysfunction, tubal pelvic factors, immune factors, and unexplained infertility. Recently, researches on the mechanism of infertility are mainly divided into the general influence of HPO axis, the influence of the ovary (ovarian micro-environment, oocyte quality, ovarian blood vessel, etc.), fallopian tube (inflammation, fallopian tube adhesion), or uterine cavity (anatomic anomaly, endometrium adhesion, imbalance of maternal-fetal interface, etc.). Acupuncture is an alternative auxiliary therapy for infertility, especially for COH during ovulation. Its mechanism of improving pregnancy outcomes has also attracted the attention of scientific researchers.

3.1 Influence of the HPO axis

The HPO axis plays an important role in female estrous cycle and reproduction, and its normal positive and negative feedback is the basis for ensuring normal reproductive function and promoting egg maturation, and triggering ovulation.
The secretion and release of gonadotropin-releasing hormone (GnRH) released by the hypothalamus to the pituitary portal system can be induced and controlled by the stimulation of other mediators in different brain regions [33, 34]. Various mediators such as central neurotransmitters and neuropeptides are integrated into the hypothalamus to regulate the reproductive system. The neurotransmitters norepinephrine and prostaglandin E_2 regulate the activity of hypothalamic neurons and are potential stimulators affecting the release of GnRH in the hypothalamus [35]. Zhu et al. found that electroacupuncture (EA) stimulated bilateral *Sanyinjiao* and bilateral *Zusanli*, three times a week, five sessions in total. It was found that GnRH, follicle-stimulating hormone (FSH), luteinizing hormone (LH), as well as 17 β-estradiol, progesterone (P), and norepinephrine were changed in the EA group compared with the blank or placebo group. Studies have shown that EA can regulate the homeostasis of the HPO axis in physiological rats [36].

The most common abnormalities of the HPO axis are ovulation disorders. Such as PCOS, POI, POF, etc. Stener-Victorin reported that repeated EA stimulation significantly promoted beta-endorphin release from the hypothalamus in polycystic ovary (PCO) rats and decreased nerve growth factor (NGF), corticotropin-releasing factor, and endothelin-1 in the PCO rats [37, 38]. Further studies showed that low-frequency EA with PCOS for a total of 25 sessions improved impaired endorphin dysfunction and regulated the immune system in steroid-induced PCO rats [39]. In another study, EA improved disturbed estrus cycles in adolescent PCO rats, upregulated lutein level and ovarian volume [40], and EA elevated LH, and restored reduced estradiol and GnRH.

3.2 Influence of the ovary

Ovarian tissue facilitates the maturation of ovum. Ovarian dysfunction will lead to poor development of ovum, resulting in embryo fertilization failure, which may eventually lead to poor pregnancy outcomes. Current studies have shown that ovarian dysfunction was caused by ovarian inflammation, excessive oxidative stress of ovarian interstitial cells, abnormal intestinal flora, epigenetic changes, abnormal ovarian immunity, etc. The effects of acupuncture on ovarian function through physical stimulation have been reported as follows:

During follicular development, granulosa cells are responsible for providing nutrients required maturation of the ovum. Follicular atresia and apoptosis are closely related to granulosa cell apoptosis. Acupuncture can increase the expression of B-cell lymphoma-2 (BCL-2) and reduce the expression of BCL-2 protein to reduce the apoptosis of granulosa cells, hence serving as an escort for follicular development. EA has been shown to effectively improve oocyte quality and embryo development potential in PCOS infertility patients [41]. EA has been shown to improve follicular dysplasia in PCOS patients by inhibiting overexpression of anti-Mullerian hormone (AMH) and increasing the expression of P450arom [42]. Acupuncture can improve ovulation disorder by down-regulating lnccmeg3 expression, inhibiting phosphatidylinositol 3-kinase (PI3K)/AKT/mammalian target of rapamycin (mTOR) pathway and reducing granulocyte autophagy [43].

Fat and environmental factors are strongly associated with the development of POF, and diets high in fat and sugar (HFHS) can impair ovarian function and ovum quality [44]. Recent studies have shown that acupuncture can improve ovarian damage induced by HFHS. Promote follicular maturation by inhibiting ovarian fibrosis and follicular atresia [45]. Moreover, the study found that it was mainly related to inhibiting ovarian oxidative stress and Fe2+ accumulation in modeled rats, and further exploration found that it may be related to affecting intestinal flora changes.

3.3 Influence of the endometrium

Endometrium is the soil for successful embryo implantation. At present, ART technology has obtained relatively good-quality embryos, nevertheless, the implantation rate remains low. Among them, the poor implantation environment of embryos caused by abnormal endometrium is the focus of attention. Among them, an abnormal intimal environment, including abnormal intimal blood flow, leads to low receptivity and decreased ability to accept embryos, leading to recurrent implantation failure (RIF). Or the imbalanced intimal immunity may lead to the disturbance of the maternal-fetal immune interface and affect the embryo implantation window (WOI). The research showed that acupuncture treatment significantly repaired endometrium dysfunction, especially caused by COH.

3.3.1 Balance between the window of implantation and embryo after ovarian hyperstimulation

Studies have demonstrated that COH-induced hyper-physiological levels of estrogen and progesterone, high progesterone ratio, unbalance of glycosyl coupling, or imbalance of human chorionic gonadotropin (HCG) administrated rats. COH procedure may lead to endometrial dysplasia, endometrial and embryonic dysplasia, and affect angiogenesis, leading to implantation failure [46]. Many cytokines are involved in the regulation of angiogenesis in the endometrium, including vascular endothelial growth factor (VEGF), fibroblast growth factor (FGF), and the angiopoietin family [47, 48]. Dong et al. Established a rat model of COH by injecting serum gonadotropin (PMSG) and HCG into pregnant mares. The rats were treated with EA from the day of PMSG injection to the third day of gestation. The results showed that the endometrial VEGF content and endometrial dendritic cells (DCs) were affected while the patient was in the peri-implantation phase. It was found that acupuncture combined with progesterone could improve endometrial VEGF and regulate DCs to promote implantation [49]. The team further found that EA promoted the implantation of COH rat embryos by activating the VEGFR2/PI3K/AKT and VEGFR2/ERK signaling pathways, which are positively correlated with endometrial angiogenesis [50]. A recent study conducted by the team, a scanning electron microscope on the rat endometrium after COH. The pinopodes of the endometrium tissues were observed after ovarian retrieval, after four days, five days, and six days by a microscope, respectively, and found that the pinopodes were distributed in advance after COH. atrophy and subside in advance, and the acupuncture treatment group can significantly pull back the forward movement of pinopodes. Thus, EA can synchronize embryo implantation and endometrial acceptance, and restore timely WOI. [21].

You et al. also found that acupuncture could improve endometrial acceptance after COH, and low-frequency acupuncture (2 Hz, 1 mA, 20 min) and high-frequency acupuncture (50 Hz, 1 mA, 20 min) were administrated in *Guanyuan* and *Zusanli*, respectively. High-frequency EA significantly decreased the protein expression levels of E-cadherin, β-catenin, and CLDN1 adhesion molecules after the COH procedure, and significantly enhanced the LIF/ STAT3 signaling pathway [51], LIF promoted cell transplantation, differentiation, and regulated endometrial receptivity. Moreover, LIF regulates phosphorylation of STAT3 and affects embryo implantation in the endometrium [52]. The team further found that EA promoted the expression of LIF/ STAT3 signals by inhibiting miR-223-3p, thereby enhancing the expression of endometrial adhesion proteins (E-cadherin, β-catenin, and CLDN1 adhesion molecules) to successful embryo implantation [53].

In conclusion, COH increases the content of serum estrogen and progesterone, regulates the hormone receptors on the endometrium, and thus affects WOI, resulting in the failure of embryo implantation. However, acupuncture/EA during COH can synchronize WOI with embryonic development and improve the rate of embryo implantation while improving the quantity and quality of embryos. And high-frequency EA has more advantages than low-frequency EA.

3.3.2 Improvement of the endometrium morphology

Normal endometrial morphology is the key factor of embryo implantation, including endometrial thickness, endometrial typing, sub-endometrial blood flow, etc. Excessive curettage, endocrine disruption, and endometrial tuberculosis would lead to thinning of the endometrial and limited growth. Thin endometrium may also be caused by dysplasia of the basal vessels of the endometrium. Thin endometrium has an impact on female fertility, resulting in low implantation rates and high miscarriage rates [54]. It has been shown that EA combined with bone marrow mesenchymal stem cells (BMSC) can improve the thickness of thin endometrial rats molded with 95% ethanol, and EA promotes migration of transplanted BMSCs to the damaged uterus by activating the stromal cell-derived faction-1/C-X-C chemokine receptor 4 (SDF-1/ CXCR4) axis. It was also found that the secretion of VEGF and basic fibroblast growth factor (bFGF) in endometrial lesions increased, and the implantation rate of embryos increased. Therefore, it is suggested that EA plays an important role in supporting BMSCs to repair thin endometrium, possibly by promoting the migration of BMSCs and enhancing the paracrine effect of bone marrow mesenchymal stem cells [55].

3.3.3 Equilibrium of the maternal-fetal immune interface

Immune cells located at the interface between the placenta and uterus are thought to play an important role in successful pregnancy. Recent studies have shown that the composition and function of these cells are locally controlled by the uterine mesenchymal cell peri-implantation. Key immune cell types include: natural killer (NK) cells, macrophages, dendritic cells and T cells, and the balance of these cells determines the success of embryo implantation to varying degrees [56].

Huang et al. found that acupuncture could regulate the endometrial immune microenvironment of pregnant rats. Acupuncture in the *Zusanli* and *Sanyinjiao* rats detected that it could improve the poor reception status of the endometrium by promoting the secretion of LIF and interleukin-12 (IL-12) in the endometrium [57]. Further research found that significantly reduced implanted embryos after mifepristone modeling, while acupuncture and progesterone treatment could significantly improve the implantation. Mifepristone significantly decreased the expression of CCL2 and CXCL8 protein and mRNA, and acupuncture or progesterone significantly reversed the expression of CCL2 and CXCL8 protein and mRNA. Acupuncture with progesterone significantly increased uterine natural killer (uNK) cell subsets in rats with failed implantation [58]. Further studies showed that acupuncture promoted implantation and placenta formation in embryonic rats by improving the expression of CXCR1 and CXCR2 at the maternal-fetal boundary [59].

4. Mechanism of acupuncture treatment of male infertility

Male infertility is one of the most common diseases in andrology, which accounts for about half of the incidence of infertility in couples. Some male diseases such as oligospermia, asthenospermia, azoospermia, and others may be some of the common factors leading to male infertility. IVF-ET, ICSI, and intrauterine insemination (IUI) are important methods for male infertility in ART. However, the success rate of ART remained unsatisfactory due to various factors, and the evaluation of the male was often neglected. By optimizing male fertility, couples are able to choose less invasive ART techniques and/or enhance ART outcomes. In recent years, acupuncture, as the non-pharmacological therapy of traditional Chinese medicine with the advantages of significant efficacy and few adverse effects, has been increasingly accepted in the treatment of male infertility. The efficacy and possible mechanisms of acupuncture for male infertility are described below to provide a basis for the treatment of male infertility with acupuncture.

4.1 Acupuncture improves sperm parameters

The male sperm factor is an important aspect of pregnancy failure. Impaired sperm parameters such as semen volume, sperm concentration, sperm motility, and total sperm count are closely associated with conception and embryo quality [60, 61]. A retrospective, real-world study demonstrated that progressive sperm motility was the main ART outcomes predictor for the frozen cycle, which need to be improved for ART success [62]. Recently, a Bayesian network meta-analysis found that EA can effectively improve sperm motility [63]. In addition, spermatozoa morphology is also an important indicator of male sperm quality. A decline in normal spermatozoa morphology may reduce pregnancy rates and affect the outcome of ART [64]. Gurfinkel et al. found that the ratio of normal-form sperm in patients with semen abnormalities was significantly increased after acupuncture and moxibustion treatments [65].

Acupuncture could increase the blood flow of the testis and provide a suitable internal environment for spermatogenesis. A prospective, randomized study [66] found that 10 Hz EA stimulation resulted in a significant increase in testicular artery parameters in volume flow, end-diastolic velocity, PSV, diameter, and area. The mechanism may be related to the testicular sympathetic reflex response controlled by the supraspinal pathway. Siterman et al. [67] found an increase in sperm concentration and a reduction in local testicular temperature to normal levels after acupuncture treatment in oligozoospermia caused by inflammation of the reproductive tract. Immune factors are another important cause of male infertility, which may be caused by antisperm antibodies (AsAb), that is immune infertility [68]. A clinical report pointed out that the positive rate of AsAb decreased significantly after the treatment of acupuncture combined with herbal drugs, and the curative effect was better than that of oral prednisone [69].

4.2 Regulation mechanism of sperm quality by acupuncture

Sperm quality is an important aspect of pregnancy failure. The sperm parameters, such as semen volume, sperm concentration, sperm motility, and total sperm count, are closely associated with conception and embryo quality, and impaired sperm parameters may reduce pregnancy rates and affect the outcome of ART. With the increasing acceptance of acupuncture in ART procedures, several studies have demonstrated the effect of acupuncture in improving sperm quality, and research on the related mechanisms has been gradually conducted. In recent years, oxidative stress which affects semen parameters has gradually attracted attention in the pathogenesis of male infertility [70]. And the sperm CatSper channel was essential for male fertility [71] and the endocrine system plays an important role in the regulation of male sperm parameters [72]. Accumulated evidence showed the potential of acupuncture in the improvement of sperm quality by regulating oxidative stress [71], sperm CatSper channels, and the hypothalamic–pituitary-gonadal axis which may be the related mechanism of acupuncture for male infertility.

4.2.1 Acupuncture regulates sperm anti-oxidative stress pathway

Particularly, EA combines the benefits of electrical stimulation and traditional acupuncture therapy, which could regulate the oxidative stress pathway and reduce oxidative stress injury. In order to observe the effect of EA on the antioxidant function of Leydig cells in aged rats with low T levels, the study found that the levels of serum total testosterone (TT) and free testosterone (FT) and the expressions of phosphorylated extracellular signal-regulated protein kinase (p-ERK), ERK, nuclear factor erythroid 2-related factor 2 (Nrf2) and heme oxy-genase-1 (HO-1) proteins in

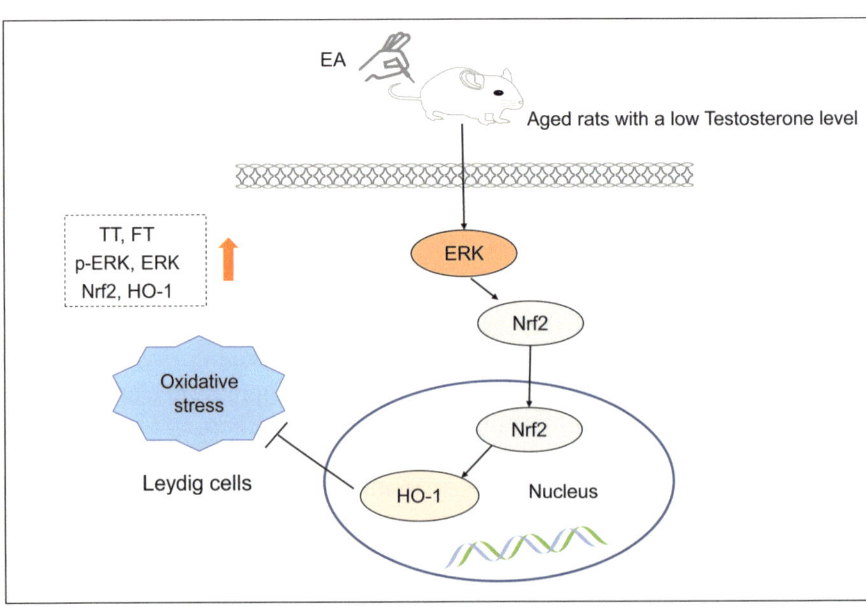

Figure 2.
EA regulates the anti-oxidative stress pathway of ERK/Nrf2/HO-1 [73]. Abbreviation: TT, total testosterone; FT, free testosterone; p-ERK, phosphorylated extracellular signal-regulated protein kinase; Nrf2, nuclear factor erythroid 2-related factor 2; HO-1, heme oxy-genase-1; EA, electroacupuncture.

the testis were significantly increased after EA treatment, which may be related to the regulation of the anti-oxidative stress pathway of ERK/Nrf2/HO-1 and the reduction of oxidative stress injury by EA to improve the reproductive function **Figure 2** [73].

4.2.2 Acupuncture regulates sperm CatSper channels

CatSper channel, a sperm-specific calcium channel including four pore-forming α subunits (CatSper1-CatSper4), was essential for the regulation of sperm motility, hyperactivity, and male fertility [71, 74]. The abundance of CatSper protein was significantly decreased in sperm of idiopathic asthenozoospermia (iAZS) patients. The result of animal experiment showed that the sperm motility of idiopathic asthenozoospermia rats was improved after EA treatment. In particular, 2 Hz-EA treatment can reverse the decreased protein tyrosine phosphorylation, over-activation, acrosome reaction, and other sperm dysfunction and fertility impairment in AZS rats. The possible mechanism may be associated with that 2 Hz TEAS or EA treatment enhanced the functional expression of CatSper channels in the sperm [11]. In addition, an RCT demonstrated that the sperm count and motility in patients with abnormal semen parameters were improved after 2 months of treatment of TEAS, which may be related to the increase of zinc, Neutral α-glucosidase and fructose levels in seminal plasma and the regulation of calcium-and integrin-binding protein-1 (CIB1) and cyclin-dependent kinase 1 (CDK1) (**Figure 3**) [75].

4.2.3 Acupuncture regulates the hypothalamic: Pituitary-gonadal axis

The endocrine system plays an important role in maintaining normal reproductive function. The spermatogenesis was regulated by the hypothalamic–pituitary-gonadal

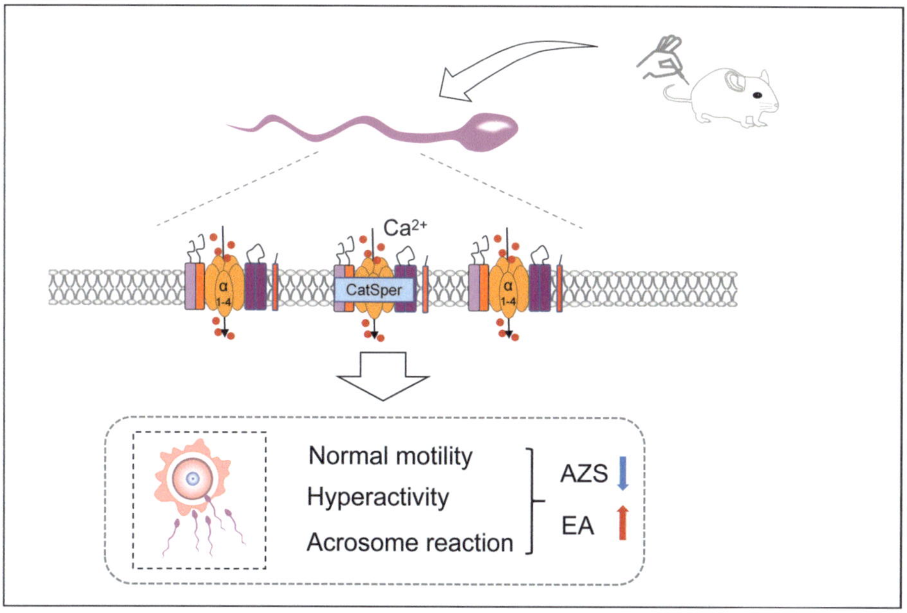

Figure 3.
Mechanism of EA in the treatment of asthenospermia through the CatSper pathway [11]. Abbreviation: EA, electroacupuncture; iAZS, idiopathic asthenozoospermia.

axis [72]. The hypothalamus synthesizes and secretes GnRH to stimulate the pituitary, which produces FSH and LH to act on testes and regulate the endocrine and spermatogenic processes [76]. Abnormal FSH and LH levels decreased testosterone synthesis, which is required for the spermatogenic cycle and plays an integral role in spermatogenesis, sperm maturation, and sperm release, resulting in decreased fertility and even infertility. A systematic review and meta-analysis demonstrated that 2 Hz transcutaneous electrical acupoint stimulation (TEAS) and EA were effective in improving the reproductive hormones FSH, LH, and testosterone in Oligoasthenospermia patients [63]. Cao et al. conducted an animal experiment and found that acupuncture reduced the LH level and increased the testosterone level and sperm density and motility in rats with oligoasthenospermia [77].

5. Summary and outlook

Over the past two decades, acupuncture has played a significant and increasingly recognized role in supporting and enhancing various assisted reproductive techniques. Acupuncture holds promising prospects as a complementary therapy in the field of assisted reproductive technology, offering potential improvements in reproductive outcomes, emotional well-being, and overall patient experiences. By incorporating acupuncture into routine practice, individuals undergoing assisted reproductive treatments have the opportunity to enhance their chances of success and overall satisfaction.

Acupuncture serves as a valuable aid in reproductive technology by targeting specific acupuncture points and meridians that are closely associated with reproductive function. Skilled acupuncturists utilize techniques such as needling, moxibustion, and acupressure to stimulate these points, restoring the body's energy balance. This holistic approach aims to optimize the reproductive system, improve the quality of eggs and sperm, regulate menstrual cycles, enhance uterine receptivity, and support the implantation process.

The development of acupuncture-assisted reproductive technology has been a gradual process, with research studies and clinical trials providing evidence of its potential benefits. However, it is important to note that further high-quality research is needed to consolidate these findings and provide stronger support. Continued exploration of acupuncture's mechanisms of action, refinement of treatment protocols, and larger-scale clinical trials will contribute to a better understanding of its efficacy and enable its optimal integration into standard assisted reproductive technology protocols.

Conflict of interest

The authors declare no conflict of interest.

Abbreviations

IVF	*In vitro* fertilization
ART	assisted reproductive technology
AI	artificial insemination
IVF-ET	in vitro fertilization-embryo transfer
CPR	clinical pregnancy rate

LBR	live birth rate
EA	electroacupuncture
HPO	hypothalamic–pituitary-ovarian
COH	controlled ovarian hyperstimulation
OHSS	ovarian hyperstimulation syndrome
POR	poor ovarian response
UBF	uterine blood flow
PCOS	polycystic ovary syndrome
POI	poor ovarian insufficient
POF	premature ovarian failure
DOR	diminished ovarian reserve
OBF	ovary blood flow
PSV	peak systolic velocity
ICSI	intracytoplasmic sperm injection
OPR	ongoing pregnancy rate
FET	frozen embryo transfer
GnRH	gonadotropin-releasing hormone
FSH	follicle-stimulating hormone
LH	luteinizing hormone
PCO	hypothalamus in polycystic ovary
NGF	nerve growth factor
BCL-2	B-cell lymphoma-2
AMH	anti-Mullerian hormone
PI3K	phosphatidylinositol 3-kinase
mTOR	mammalian target of rapamycin
HFHS	high in fat and sugar
RIF	recurrent implantation failure
WOI	embryo implantation window
HCG	human chorionic gonadotropin
VEGF	vascular endothelial growth factor
FGF	fibroblast growth factor
PMSG	serum gonadotropin
DCs	dendritic cells
BMSC	bone marrow mesenchymal stem cells
SDF-1	stromal cell derived faction-1
CXCR4	C-X-C chemokine receptor 4
bFGF	basic fibroblast growth factor
NK	natural killer
IL-12	interleukin-12
uNK	uterine natural killer
AsAb	antisperm antibodies
TT	total testosterone
FT	free testosterone
p-ERK	phosphorylated extracellular signal-regulated protein kinase
Nrf2	nuclear factor erythroid 2-related factor 2
HO-1	heme oxy-genase-1
iAZS	idiopathic asthenozoospermia
CIB1	calcium-and integrin-binding protein-1
CDK1	cyclin-dependent kinase 1
TEAS	transcutaneous electrical acupoint stimulation

Author details

Jie Yang[1], Liying Liu[1,2], Xiaoyan Zheng[1], Jingwen Zhang[1] and Yuanyuan Lai[1,2]*

1 Acupuncture and Tuina School, Chengdu University of Traditional Chinese Medicine, Chengdu, China

2 Sichuan Jinxin Xi'nan Women's and Children's Hospital, Chengdu, China

*Address all correspondence to: jenny_yang_jie@126.com

References

[1] Carson SA, Kallen AN. Diagnosis and Management of Infertility: A review. Journal of the American Medical Association. 2021;**326**(1):65-76. DOI: 10.1001/jama.2021.4788

[2] Vander, Borght M, Wyns C. Fertility and infertility: Definition and epidemiology. Clinical Biochemistry. Dec 2018;**62**:2-10. DOI: 10.1016/j.clinbiochem.2018.03.012. PMID: 29555319

[3] Graham ME, Jelin A, Hoon AH, Wilms Floet AM, Levey E, Graham EM. Assisted reproductive technology: Short- and long-term outcomes. Developmental Medicine and Child Neurology. 2023;**65**(1):38-49. DOI: 10.1111/dmcn.15332

[4] Fishel S. First in vitro fertilization baby-this is how it happened. Fertility and Sterility. Jul 1 2018;**110**(1):5-11. DOI: 10.1016/j.fertnstert.2018.03.008. Epub 2018 Jun 13. PMID: 29908772

[5] Berntsen S, Söderström-Anttila V, Wennerholm U-B, Laivuori H, Loft A, Oldereid NB, et al. The health of children conceived by ART: 'the chicken or the egg?'. Human Reproduction Update. 2019;**25**(2):137-158. DOI: 10.1093/humupd/dmz001

[6] Roque M, Haahr T, Geber S, Esteves SC, Humaidan P. Fresh versus elective frozen embryo transfer in IVF/ICSI cycles: A systematic review and meta-analysis of reproductive outcomes. Human Reproduction Update. Jan 1 2019;**25**(1):2-14. DOI: 10.1093/humupd/dmy033. PMID: 30388233

[7] Calhaz-Jorge C, De Geyter C, Kupka MS, de Mouzon J, Erb K, Mocanu E, et al. Assisted reproductive technology in Europe, 2013: Results generated from European registers by ESHRE. Human Reproduction (Oxford, England). 2017;**32**(10):1957-1973. DOI: 10.1093/humrep/dex264

[8] Gunby J, Bissonnette F, Librach C, Cowan L. IVF Directors Group of the Canadian Fertility and Andrology Society. Assisted reproductive technologies (ART) in Canada: 2007 results from the Canadian ART register. Fertility and Sterility. 2011;**95**(2):542-7.e1-10. DOI: 10.1016/j.fertnstert.2010.05.057. pub 2010 Jul 24. PMID: 20656287

[9] Stener-Victorin E, Waldenström U, Nilsson L, Wikland M, Janson PO. A prospective randomized study of electro-acupuncture versus alfentanil as anaesthesia during oocyte aspiration in in-vitro fertilization. Human Reproduction. 1999;**14**(10):2480-2484. DOI: 10.1093/humrep/14.10.2480

[10] Xi J, Pan Y, Jin C, Liu J, Cheng J, Xu B. Evaluation of different rat models intrauterine adhesion models and improvement of the technique for their establishment. Experimental Animals. May 17;**72**(2):274-284. DOI: 10.1538/expanim.22-0153. PMID: 36642541; PMCID: PMC10202710

[11] Jin ZR, Fang D, Liu BH, Cai J, Tang WH, Jiang H, et al. Roles of CatSper channels in the pathogenesis of asthenozoospermia and the therapeutic effects of acupuncture-like treatment on asthenozoospermia. Theranostics. 2021;**11**(6):2822-2844

[12] Magarelli PC, Cridennda DK, Cohen M. Changes in serum cortisol and prolactin associated with acupuncture during controlled ovarian hyperstimulation in women undergoing

in vitro fertilization-embryo transfer treatment. Fertility and Sterility. 2009;**92**(6):1870-1879. DOI: 10.1016/j.fertnstert.2008.10.067

[13] Ferraretti AP, La Marca A, Fauser BC, Tarlatzis B, Nargund G, Gianaroli L, et al. ESHRE consensus on the definition of 'poor response' to ovarian stimulation for in vitro fertilization: The Bologna criteria. Human Reproduction. 2011;**26**(7):1616-1624. DOI: 10.1093/humrep/der092

[14] Wang RR, Su MH, Liu LY, Lai YY, Guo XL, Gan D, et al. Systematic review of acupuncture to improve ovarian function in women with poor ovarian response. Frontiers in Endocrinology. 2023;**14**:1028853. DOI: 10.3389/fendo.2023.1028853

[15] Kim J, Lee H, Choi TY, Kim JI, Kang BK, Lee MS, et al. Acupuncture for poor ovarian response: A randomized controlled trial. Journal of Clinical Medicine. May 18 2021;**10**(10):2182. DOI: 10.3390/jcm10102182. PMID: 34070086; PMCID: PMC8158119

[16] Battaglia C. The role of ultrasound and Doppler analysis in the diagnosis of polycystic ovary syndrome. Ultrasound in Obstetrics & Gynecology. 2003;**22**(3):225-232. DOI: 10.1002/uog.228

[17] Wang WQ, Chu GH, Hou XX. A comparison of Doppler measures of ovarian blood flow between women with and without ovarian dysfunction and correlations of Doppler indices with ovarian dysfunction markers: A meta-analysis. Annals of Translational Medicine. 2023;**11**(2):110. DOI: 10.21037/atm-22-5813

[18] Zampini EG, Gallelli MF, Chaves MG, Neild DM, Gambarotta M, Miragaya MH, et al. Uterine and Corpus luteum blood flow evaluation prior to uterine Flushing in llama embryo donors. Frontiers in Veterinary Science. 2020;**7**:597960. DOI: 10.3389/fvets.2020.597960

[19] Ng EH, So WS, Gao J, Wong YY, Ho PC. The role of acupuncture in the management of subfertility. Fertility and Sterility. 2008;**90**(1):1-13. DOI: 10.1016/j.fertnstert.2008.02.094

[20] Zheng X, Yu S, Liu L, Yang H, Wang F, Yang H, et al. The dose-related efficacy of acupuncture on endometrial receptivity in infertile women: A systematic review and Meta-analysis. Frontiers in Public Health. 2022;**10**:858587. DOI: 10.3389/fpubh.2022.858587

[21] Hu R, Huang Y, Song Y, Wu X, Song K, Huang G, et al. Effect of acupuncture on the opening time of implantation window and endometrial receptivity in controlled ovarian hyperstimulation rats during peri-implantation period. Frontiers in Endocrinology. 2023;**14**:1110266. DOI: 10.3389/fendo.2023.1110266

[22] Zhong Y, Zeng F, Liu W, Ma J, Guan Y, Song Y. Acupuncture in improving endometrial receptivity: A systematic review and meta-analysis. BMC Complementary and Alternative Medicine. 2019;**19**(1):61. DOI: 10.1186/s12906-019-2472-1

[23] Jo J, Lee YJ. Effectiveness of acupuncture in women with polycystic ovarian syndrome undergoing in vitro fertilisation or intracytoplasmic sperm injection: A systematic review and meta-analysis. Acupuncture in Medicine. 2017;**35**(3):162-170. DOI: 10.1136/acupmed-2016-011163

[24] Turner K, Reynolds-May MF, Zitek EM, Tisdale RL, Carlisle AB,

Westphal LM. Stress and anxiety scores in first and repeat IVF cycles: A pilot study. PLoS One. 2013;**8**(5):e63743. DOI: 10.1371/journal.pone.0063743

[25] Hullender Rubin LE, Smith CA, Schnyer RN, Tahir P, Pasch LA. Effect of acupuncture on IVF-related anxiety: A systematic review and meta-analysis. Reproductive Biomedicine Online. 2022;**45**(1):69-80. DOI: 10.1016/j.rbmo.2022.02.002

[26] Liu LY, Tian ZL, Zhu FT, Yang H, Xiao F, Wang RR, et al. Systematic review and Meta-analysis of acupuncture for pain Management in Women Undergoing Transvaginal Oocyte Retrieval. Journal of Pain Research. 2021;**14**:2833-2849. DOI: 10.2147/jpr.S319923

[27] Humaidan P, Brock K, Bungum L, Stener-Victorin E. Pain relief during oocyte retrieval--exploring the role of different frequencies of electro-acupuncture. Reproductive Biomedicine Online. 2006;**13**(1):120-125. DOI: 10.1016/s1472-6483(10)62025-1

[28] Stener-Victorin E. The pain-relieving effect of electro-acupuncture and conventional medical analgesic methods during oocyte retrieval: A systematic review of randomized controlled trials. Human Reproduction. 2005;**20**(2):339-349. DOI: 10.1093/humrep/deh595

[29] Smith CA, de Lacey S, Chapman M, Ratcliffe J, Norman RJ, Johnson NP, et al. Effect of acupuncture vs sham acupuncture on live births among women undergoing In vitro fertilization: A randomized clinical trial. Journal of the American Medical Association. 2018;**319**(19):1990-1998. DOI: 10.1001/jama.2018.5336

[30] Manheimer E, van der Windt D, Cheng K, Stafford K, Liu J, Tierney J, et al. The effects of acupuncture on rates of clinical pregnancy among women undergoing in vitro fertilization: A systematic review and meta-analysis. Human Reproduction Update. 2013;**19**(6):696-713. DOI: 10.1093/humupd/dmt026

[31] Zheng CH, Huang GY, Zhang MM, Wang W. Effects of acupuncture on pregnancy rates in women undergoing in vitro fertilization: A systematic review and meta-analysis. Fertility and Sterility. 2012;**97**(3):599-611. DOI: 10.1016/j.fertnstert.2011.12.007

[32] Zhu C, Xia W, Huang J, Zhang X, Li F, Yu X, et al. Effects of acupuncture on the pregnancy outcomes of frozen-thawed embryo transfer: A systematic review and meta-analysis. Frontiers in Public Health. 2022;**10**:987276. DOI: 10.3389/fpubh.2022.987276

[33] Moore AM, Abbott G, Mair J, Prescott M, Campbell RE. Mapping GABA and glutamate inputs to gonadotrophin-releasing hormone neurones in male and female mice. Journal of Neuroendocrinology. 2018;**30**(12):e12657. DOI: 10.1111/jne.12657

[34] Saedi S, Khoradmehr A, Mohammad Reza JS, Tamadon A. The role of neuropeptides and neurotransmitters on kisspeptin/kiss1r-signaling in female reproduction. Journal of Chemical Neuroanatomy. 2018;**92**:71-82. DOI: 10.1016/j.jchemneu.2018.07.001

[35] Fujioka H, Funabashi T, Akema T. Prostaglandin E2 modulates presynaptic regulation of GnRH neurons via EP4 receptors in accordance with estrogen milieu. Neuroscience. 2017;**360**:139-145. DOI: 10.1016/j.neuroscience.2017.07.025

[36] Zhu H, Nan S, Suo C, Zhang Q, Hu M, Chen R, et al. Electro-acupuncture affects the activity of the hypothalamic-pituitary-ovary Axis in female rats.

Frontiers in Physiology. 2019;**10**:466. DOI: 10.3389/fphys.2019.00466

[37] Stener-Victorin E, Lundeberg T, Waldenström U, Bileviciute-Ljungar I, Janson PO. Effects of electro-acupuncture on corticotropin-releasing factor in rats with experimentally-induced polycystic ovaries. Neuropeptides. 2001;**35**(5-6):227-231. DOI: 10.1054/npep.2002.0878

[38] Stener-Victorin E, Lundeberg T, Cajander S, Aloe L, Manni L, Waldenström U, et al. Steroid-induced polycystic ovaries in rats: Effect of electro-acupuncture on concentrations of endothelin-1 and nerve growth factor (NGF), and expression of NGF mRNA in the ovaries, the adrenal glands, and the central nervous system. Reproductive Biology and Endocrinology: RB&E. 2003;**1**:33. DOI: 10.1186/1477-7827-1-33

[39] Stener-Victorin E, Lindholm C. Immunity and beta-endorphin concentrations in hypothalamus and plasma in rats with steroid-induced polycystic ovaries: Effect of low-frequency electroacupuncture. Biology of Reproduction. 2004;**70**(2):329-333. DOI: 10.1095/biolreprod.103.022368

[40] Wang Z, Yang L, Dong H, Dong H, Cheng L, Yi P, et al. Effect of electroacupuncture on the kisspeptin system in a pubertal rat model of polycystic ovary syndrome. Acupuncture in Medicine : Journal of the British Medical Acupuncture Society. 2021;**39**(5):491-500. DOI: 10.1177/0964528420971299

[41] Xiang S, Xia MF, Song JY, Liu DQ, Lian F. Effect of electro-acupuncture on expression of IRS-1/PI3K/GLUT4 pathway in ovarian granulosa cells of infertile patients with polycystic ovary syndrome-insulin resistance of phlegm-dampness syndrome. Chinese Journal of Integrative Medicine. 2021;**27**(5):330-335. DOI: 10.1007/s11655-020-3219-z

[42] Zhao QY, Sun Y, Zhou J, Gao YL, Ma GZ, Hu ZH, et al. Effectiveness of herb-partitioned moxibustion combined with electroacupuncture on polycystic ovary syndrome in patients with symptom pattern of kidney deficiency and phlegm-dampne. Journal of Traditional Chinese Medicine = Chung i tsa chih ying wen pan. 2021;**41**(6):985-993. DOI: 10.19852/j.cnki.jtcm.2021.06.017

[43] Chen X, Tang H, Liang Y, Wu P, Xie L, Ding Y, et al. Acupuncture regulates the autophagy of ovarian granulosa cells in polycystic ovarian syndrome ovulation disorder by inhibiting the PI3K/AKT/mTOR pathway through LncMEG3. Biomedicine & Pharmacotherapy = Biomedecine & Pharmacotherapie. 2021;**144**:112288. DOI: 10.1016/j.biopha.2021.112288

[44] Wang N, Luo LL, Xu JJ, Xu MY, Zhang XM, Zhou XL, et al. Obesity accelerates ovarian follicle development and follicle loss in rats. Metabolism: Clinical and Experimental. 2014;**63**(1):94-103. DOI: 10.1016/j.metabol.2013.09.001

[45] Geng Z, Nie X, Ling L, Li B, Liu P, Yuan L, et al. Electroacupuncture May inhibit oxidative stress of premature ovarian failure mice by regulating intestinal microbiota. Oxidative Medicine and Cellular Longevity. 2022;**2022**:4362317. DOI: 10.1155/2022/4362317

[46] Kliman HJ, Frankfurter D. Clinical approach to recurrent implantation failure: Evidence-based evaluation of the endometrium. Fertility and Sterility. 2019;**111**(4):618-628. DOI: 10.1016/j.fertnstert.2019.02.011

[47] Smith SK. Regulation of angiogenesis in the endometrium. Trends in Endocrinology and Metabolism: TEM. 2001;**12**(4):147-151. DOI: 10.1016/s1043-2760(01)00379-4

[48] Rizov M, Andreeva P, Dimova I. Molecular regulation and role of angiogenesis in reproduction. Taiwanese Journal of Obstetrics & Gynecology. 2017;**56**(2):127-132. DOI: 10.1016/j.tjog.2016.06.019

[49] Dong H, Zhong Z, Chen W, Wu X, Zhang Q, Huang G, et al. Effect of acupuncture on endometrial angiogenesis and uterus dendritic cells in COH rats during Peri-implantation period. Evidence-Based Complementary and Alternative Medicine : eCAM. 2017;**2017**:3647080. DOI: 10.1155/2017/3647080

[50] Chen W, Chen J, Xu M, Zhong Z, Zhang Q, Yang W, et al. Electroacupuncture facilitates implantation by enhancing endometrial angiogenesis in a rat model of ovarian hyperstimulation. Biology of Reproduction. 2019;**100**(1):268-280. DOI: 10.1093/biolre/ioy176

[51] You F, Du X, Zhang T, Wang Y, Lv Y, Zeng L. High-frequency electroacupuncture improves endometrial receptivity via regulating cell adhesion molecules and leukemia inhibitory factor / signal transducer and activator of transcription signaling pathway. Bioengineered. 2021;**12**(2):10470-10479. DOI: 10.1080/21655979.2021.1997367

[52] Sun X, Bartos A, Whitsett JA, Dey SK. Uterine deletion of Gp130 or Stat3 shows implantation failure with increased estrogenic responses. Molecular Endocrinology (Baltimore, MD). 2013;**27**(9):1492-1501. DOI: 10.1210/me.2013-1086

[53] You F, Du X, Zhang T, Wang Y, Lv Y, Zeng L. Electroacupuncture improves endometrial receptivity through miRNA-223-3p-mediated regulation of leukemia inhibitory factor / signal transducer and activator of transcription 3 signaling pathway. Bioengineered. 2022;**13**(4):10298-10312. DOI: 10.1080/21655979.2022.2062524

[54] Shufaro Y, Simon A, Laufer N, Fatum M. Thin unresponsive endometrium--a possible complication of surgical curettage compromising ART outcome. Journal of Assisted Reproduction and Genetics. 2008;**25**(8):421-425. DOI: 10.1007/s10815-008-9245-y

[55] Xia L, Meng Q, Xi J, Han Q, Cheng J, Shen J, et al. The synergistic effect of electroacupuncture and bone mesenchymal stem cell transplantation on repairing thin endometrial injury in rats. Stem Cell Research & Therapy. 2019;**10**(1):244. DOI: 10.1186/s13287-019-1326-6

[56] Erlebacher A. Immunology of the maternal-fetal interface. Annual Review of Immunology. 2013;**31**:387-411. DOI: 10.1146/annurev-immunol-032712-100003

[57] Gui J, Xiong F, Yang W, Li J, Huang G. Effects of acupuncture on LIF and IL-12 in rats of implantation failure. American Journal of Reproductive Immunology (New York, NY: 1989). 2012;**67**(5):383-390. DOI: 10.1111/j.1600-0897.2011.01097.x

[58] Gao W, Tang X, Chen Z, Guo Y, Wang L, Zhang M, et al. Effects of acupuncture on CCL2 and CXCL8 expression and the subset of uNK cells in rats with embryo implantation failure. Evidence-Based Complementary and Alternative

Medicine : eCAM. 2013;**2013**:678390. DOI: 10.1155/2013/678390

[59] Gao WN, Yang W, Liu YF, Tang X, Guo Y, Wang LJ, et al. Effect of acupuncture on CXCL8 receptors in rats suffering from embryo implantation failure. Journal of Huazhong University of Science and Technology Medical sciences = Hua zhong ke ji da xue bao Yi xue Ying De wen ban = Huazhong keji daxue xuebao Yixue Yingdewen ban. 2014;**34**(1):91-98. DOI: 10.1007/s11596-014-1237-9

[60] Eisenberg ML, Li S, Behr B, Cullen MR, Galusha D, Lamb DJ, et al. Semen quality, infertility and mortality in the USA. Human Reproduction. 2014;**29**(7):1567-1574

[61] Jensen TK, Jacobsen R, Christensen K, Nielsen NC, Bostofte E. Good semen quality and life expectancy: A cohort study of 43,277 men. American Journal of Epidemiology. 2009;**170**(5):559-565

[62] Santi D, Spaggiari G, Morini D, Melli B, Dalla VL, Aguzzoli L, et al. Which sperm parameter limits could really guide the clinical decision in assisted reproduction? Andrology. 2023;**11**(1):143-154

[63] Wang Z, Zhou Z, Zhang L, Li X, Li M, Pan Y, et al. Efficacy and safety of nonpharmacological strategies for the treatment of oligoasthenospermia: A systematic review and Bayesian network meta-analysis. European Journal of Medical Research. 2023;**28**(1):6

[64] Palermo G, Joris H, Devroey P, Van Steirteghem AC. Pregnancies after intracytoplasmic injection of single spermatozoon into an oocyte. Lancet. 1992;**340**(8810):17-18

[65] Gurfinkel E, Cedenho AP, Yamamura Y, Srougi M. Effects of acupuncture and moxa treatment in patients with semen abnormalities. Asian Journal of Andrology. 2003;**5**(4):345-348

[66] Cakmak YO, Akpinar IN, Ekinci G, Bekiroglu N. Point- and frequency-specific response of the testicular artery to abdominal electroacupuncture in humans. Fertility and Sterility. 2008;**90**(5):1732-1738

[67] Siterman S, Eltes F, Schechter L, Maimon Y, Lederman H, Bartoov B. Success of acupuncture treatment in patients with initially low sperm output is associated with a decrease in scrotal skin temperature. Asian Journal of Andrology. 2009;**11**(2):200-208

[68] Leathersich S, Hart RJ. Immune infertility in men. Fertility and Sterility. 2022;**117**(6):1121-1131

[69] Fu B, Lun X, Gong Y. Effects of the combined therapy of acupuncture with herbal drugs on male immune infertility--a clinical report of 50 cases. Journal of Traditional Chinese Medicine. 2005;**25**(3):186-189

[70] Agarwal A, Parekh N, Panner SMK, Henkel R, Shah R, Homa ST, et al. Male oxidative stress infertility (MOSI): Proposed terminology and clinical practice guidelines for Management of Idiopathic Male Infertility. The World Journal of Men's Health. 2019;**37**(3):296-312

[71] Brown SG, Publicover SJ, Barratt CLR, Martins DSSJ. Human sperm ion channel (dys)function: Implications for fertilization. Human Reproduction Update. 2019;**25**(6):758-776

[72] Yang C, Li P, Li Z. Clinical application of aromatase inhibitors to treat male infertility. Human Reproduction Update. 2021;**28**(1):30-50

[73] Zeng TT, Yao TW, Li XZ, Tang CL. Electroacupunctureinterventionincreases testosterone level of aged rats by activating ERK/Nrf2/HO-1 signaling of Leydig cells. Zhen Ci Yan Jiu. 2019;**44**(8):566-570

[74] Lishko PV, Mannowetz N. CatSper: A unique calcium channel of the sperm flagellum. Current Opinion in Physiology. 2018;**2**:109-113

[75] Yu Y, Sha SB, Zhang B, Guan Q, Liang M, Zhao LG, et al. Effects and mechanism of action of transcutaneous electrical acupuncture point stimulation in patients with abnormal semen parameters. Acupuncture in Medicine. 2019;**37**(1):25-32

[76] Skorupskaite K, George JT, Anderson RA. The kisspeptin-GnRH pathway in human reproductive health and disease. Human Reproduction Update. 2014;**20**(4):485-500

[77] Cao YM, Jiang HZ, Li JR, Yang YP, Si JH, Ren HS, et al. Experimental study on 'Zhibian (BL54) through shuidao (ST28) 'acupuncture therapy for rats with asthenospermia and oligospermia. The Journal of Shanxi Traditional Chinese Medicine. 2021;**22**(01):26-8+32